Wound Care

made

Incredibly Easy!

Wound Care

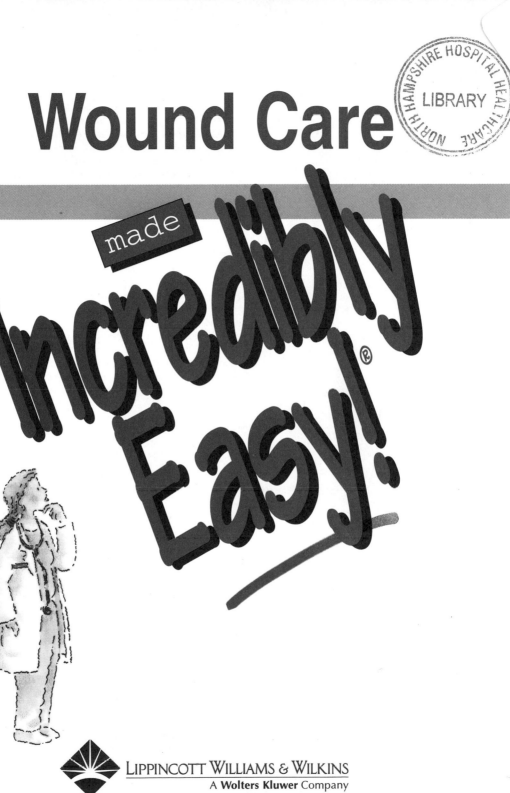

made **Incredibly Easy!**®

LIPPINCOTT WILLIAMS & WILKINS
A **Wolters Kluwer** Company

Philadelphia • Baltimore • New York • London
Buenos Aires • Hong Kong • Sydney • Tokyo

Staff

Publisher
Judith A. Schilling McCann, RN, MSN

Editorial Director
David Moreau

Clinical Director
Joan M. Robinson, RN, MSN

Senior Art Director
Arlene Putterman

Art Director
Mary Ludwicki

Clinical Project Manager
Jana Sciarra, RN, MSN, CRNP

Senior Editor
Jaime L. Stockslager

Editors
Judd Howard, Rae Theodore, Pat Wittig

Copy Editors
Kimberly Bilotta (supervisor), Scotti Cohn,
Dorothy P. Terry, Pamela Wingrod

Designers
Lynn Foulk

Illustrators
Jackie Facciolo, Judy Newhouse, Bot Roda,
Betty Winnberg

Digital Composition Services
Diane Paluba (manager), Joyce Rossi Biletz,
Richard Eng

Manufacturing
Patricia K. Dorshaw (senior manager),
Beth Janae Orr

Editorial Assistants
Danielle J. Barsky, Beverly Lane, Linda Ruhf

Indexer
Karen C. Comerford

Photo Credits
Teresa A. Conner-Kerr, PhD, PT, CWS(D);
Joan Junkin, RN, MSN, BC, CWOCN;
Mary Sieggreen, RN, MSN, CNP, CS, CVN

Library of Congress Cataloging-in-Publication Data
Wound care made incredibly easy.
   p. ; cm.
   Includes index.
   1. Wounds and injuries — Nursing.
   [DNLM: 1. Wounds and Injuries — therapy — Handbooks.
   WO 39 W938 2003] I. Lippincott Williams & Wilkins.

RD93.95.W68 2003
617.1'06—dc21
ISBN 1-58255-226-6 (pbk. : alk. paper)   2003000867

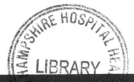

Contents

Contributors and consultants

Kathleen M. Baldwin, RN, PhD, ANP, CCRN, CEN, GNP
Associate Professor of Nursing
Texas Christian University
Fort Worth

Monica A. Beshara, RN, BSN, CWOCN
Director
Decatur-DeKalb Wound Care Center
Decatur, Ga.

Milton Derrick Boden, MD, CWS
Physician
Infectious Disease Specialists of Atlanta, PC
Decatur, Ga.

Phyllis A. Bonham, RN, MSN, CWOCN
Clinical Assistant Professor
Director, Wound Care Education Program
Medical University of South Carolina
College of Nursing
Charleston

Carol Calianno, RN, MSN, CWOCN
Wound, Ostomy, Continence Nurse
 Specialist
Abramson's Residence
North Wales, Pa.

Janice J. Clark, RN, BSN, CWOCN
ET Nurse
Wilforo Hall Medical Center
Lackland Air Force Base, Tex.

Martha D. Cobb, RN, MEd, CS, CWOCN
Clinical Associate Professor
University of Arizona College of Nursing
Tucson

Teresa A. Conner-Kerr, PhD, PT, CWS(D)
Associate Professor
East Carolina University
Greenville, N.C.

Susan M. Currence, RN, BSN, CWCN
Wound Ostomy Care Nurse
St. Joseph Medical Center
Towson, Md.

Judy A. Dutcher, MS, APRN-BC, CWOCN
Consultant
Tucson, Ariz.

Evonne M. Fowler, RN, CNS, CWOCN
Co-Director Wound Care Center
Kaiser Permanente Hospital
Bellflower, Calif.

Kelly Jaszarowski, RN, MSN, CNS, ANP, CWOCN
WOC Nurse Specialist
Central Home Health Care
Fayetteville, Ga.

Joan Junkin, RN, MSN, BC, CWOCN
Wound Ostomy Continence Coordinator
Bryan LGH Medical Center
Lincoln, Nebr.

Kim M. Kehoe, RN, BSN, CWOCN
Clinical Instructor of ET-Wound Manage-
 ment
Halifax Medical Center
Daytona Beach, Fla.

Jo Ann Maklebust, RN, MSN, CNP, CS
Nurse Practitioner
Karmanos Cancer Institute—Detroit
 Medical Center

Cammie Roy, MPT
Student PT
East Carolina University Department of
 Physical Therapy
Greenville, N.C.

Donna Scemons, RN, MSN, CNS, CWOCN, FNP
Kaiser Permanente Medical Center
Panorama City, Calif.

Mary Sieggreen, RN, MSN, CNP, CS, CVN
Nurse Practitioner, Vascular Surgery
Harper University Hospital
Detroit Medical Center

Karen Zulkowski, RN, DNS, CWS
Assistant Professor College of Nursing
Montana State University
Bozeman

Foreword

Wound care is science, not alchemy. We've come a long way from pouring sugar, applying heat lamps, and changing dressings every 2 hours. Wound care concepts and principles have changed dramatically, even since the 1970s. Yet, many clinicians still practice wound care from that era. If you're looking for the most up-to-date information on how to best care for your patients, read on because the concise, organized review of current wound care concepts in *Wound Care Made Incredibly Easy* is just what you need!

In the past decade, wound care has become an increasingly important aspect of patient care in all practice settings and specialties. Regardless of your specialty, you're bound to see various types of wounds. Chronic wounds, such as pressure ulcers and diabetic foot ulcers, are especially challenging. This indispensable reference not only tells you how these difficult wounds occur but also what you need to do to prevent and care for them.

Wound Care Made Incredibly Easy guides you through the potentially confusing maze of wound assessment (including how to classify, stage, and measure wounds as well as monitor their status), wound care planning, intervention, and wound care products. Whether you're a novice or an expert, this reference provides well-organized and succinct information that gives you confidence in your wound care decision making.

Each chapter in this one-of-a kind reference features:
• a summary of key points
• clear, simple explanations
• definitions of key terms
• an abundance of illustrations that clarify difficult concepts
• quick quizzes that help the reader assess learning.

Wound Care Made Incredibly Easy begins with the fundamentals necessary to understand and provide wound care, including a review of the integumentary system and the pathophysiology of wounds. This basic review continues with chapters on wound assessment and monitoring and wound care procedures. Each topic provides information that guides your care and treatment of wounds.

Later chapters focus on specific types of acute and chronic wounds, including surgical wounds, burns, vascular ulcers, pressure ulcers, and diabetic foot ulcers. There's even a whole chapter devoted to the therapeutic modalities currently used in wound care — from the most commonly used, such as hydrotherapy, to those still undergoing research, such as monochromatic near-infrared photo energy.

Wound care is also big business. Although the product explosion has given us many options, this proliferation of products has complicated our decision making. *Wound Care Made Incredibly Easy* addresses the dressing issue by covering the myriad of products and their correct uses.

And last but not least, this reference includes a chapter on legal and reimbursement issues, including standards of care and lots of tips that may help keep you out of court.

In addition to being well organized and easy to read and understand, *Wound Care Made Incredibly Easy* also includes these incredibly original features:

Dress for success — offers tips on wound dressings

Now I get it! — clarifies the pathophysiology of wounds and wound healing

Get wise to wounds — gives pointers on how to assess wounds, perform wound care procedures, and teach patients.

As health care professionals, we need to articulate our rationales for every wound care decision we make. *Wound Care Made Incredibly Easy* has all the information you need to provide expert care based on a solid understanding of wound care principles and practice.

Patricia A. Slachta, RN, PhD, CS, CWOCN
Chair, Division of Health Sciences
Technical College of the Low Country
Beaufort, S.C.

Wound care fundamentals

Just the facts

In this chapter, you'll learn:
♦ the layers and functions of skin
♦ the types of wounds
♦ the phases of wound healing
♦ factors that influence skin's ability to heal
♦ complications of wound healing.

A close look at the skin

The skin, or integumentary system, is the largest organ in the body. It accounts for about 6 to 8 lb (2.5 to 3.5 kg) of a person's body weight and has a surface area of more than 20 square feet. The thickest skin is located on the hands and on the soles of the feet; the thinnest skin, around the eyes and over the tympanic membranes in the ears.

The skin you're in

Skin is made up of distinct layers that function as a single unit. The outermost layer, which is actually a layer of dead cells, is completely replaced every 4 to 6 weeks by cells that migrate to the surface from the layers beneath. The living cells in the skin receive oxygen and nutrients through an extensive network of small blood vessels. In fact, every square inch of skin contains more than 15' of blood vessels!

Up close and personal

Skin protects the body by acting as a barrier between internal structures and the external world. Skin also stands between each of us and the social world around us, so it's no wonder that the condition and characteristics of a person's

> Talk about networking! Every square inch of skin contains more than 15 feet of blood vessels.

skin influence how he feels about himself. When a person has healthy skin—unblemished skin with good tone (firmness) and color—he feels better about himself. Skin also reflects the general physical health of the body. For example, if blood oxygen levels are low, skin may look bluish, and skin appears flushed or red if a person has a fever.

Be careful out there! Environmental factors such as UV radiation can wound skin.

Please Mr. Sun

Any damage to the skin is considered a wound. Wounds can result from planned events, such as surgery; accidents, such as a fall from a bike; or exposure to the environment, such as the damage caused by ultraviolet (UV) rays in sunlight.

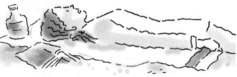

Anatomy and physiology

Skin has two main layers: the *epidermis* and *dermis*. A layer of subcutaneous fatty connective tissue, sometimes called the *hypodermis*, lies beneath these layers. Within the epidermis and dermis, which function as one interrelated unit, are five structural networks:
- collagen fibers
- elastic fibers
- small blood vessels
- nerve fibrils
- lymphatics.

These networks are stabilized by hair and sweat gland ducts.

Epidermis

The epidermis is the outermost of the skin's two main layers. It varies in thickness from about 0.1 mm thick on the eyelids to as much as 1 mm thick on the palms and soles. The epidermis is slightly acidic, with an average pH of 5.5. Covering the epidermis is the keratinized epithelium, a layer of cells that migrate up from the underlying dermis and die upon reaching the surface. These cells are continuously generated and replaced. The keratinized epithelium is supported by the dermis and underlying connective tissue.

In living color

The epidermis also contains melanocytes (cells that produce the brown pigment melanin), which give skin and hair their colors. The more melanin produced by melanocytes, the darker the skin. Skin color varies from one person to the next, but it can also vary from one area of skin on the body to another. The hypothalamus regulates melanin production by secreting melanocyte-stimulating hormone.

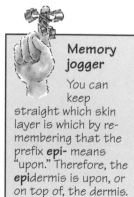

Memory jogger

You can keep straight which skin layer is which by remembering that the prefix **epi-** means "upon." Therefore, the **epi**dermis is upon, or on top of, the dermis.

Layer upon layer

The epidermis is divided into five distinct layers. Each layer's name reflects either its structure or its function. Let's look at them from the outside in:

The *stratum corneum* (horny layer) is the superficial layer of dead skin cells—the skin layer that's in contact with the environment. It has an acid mantle that helps protect the body from some fungi and bacteria. Cells in this layer are shed daily and replaced with cells from the layer beneath it, the stratum lucidum. In such diseases as eczema and psoriasis, the stratum corneum may become abnormally thick and irritate skin structures and peripheral nerves.

The *stratum lucidum* (clear layer) is a single layer of cells that forms a transitional boundary between the stratum corneum above and stratum granulosum below. This layer is most evident in areas where skin is thickest such as on the soles. It appears to be absent in areas where skin is especially thin such as on the eyelids. Although cells in this layer lack active nuclei, this is an area of intense enzyme activity that prepares cells for the stratum corneum.

The *stratum granulosum* (granular layer) is one to five cells thick and is characterized by flat cells with active nuclei. Experts believe this layer aids keratin formation.

The *stratum spinosum* is the area in which cells begin to flatten as they migrate toward the skin surface. Involucrin, a soluble protein precursor of the cornified envelopes of skin cells, is synthesized here.

The *stratum basale*, or *stratum germinativum*, is only one cell thick and is the only layer of the epidermis in which cells undergo mitosis to form new cells. The stratum basale forms the dermoepidermal junction—the area where the epidermis and dermis are connected. Protrusions of this layer (called *rete pegs* or *epidermal ridges*) extend down into the dermis where they're surrounded by vascularized dermal papillae. This unique structure supports the epidermis and facilitates the exchange of fluids and cells between the skin layers.

Dermis

The dermis—the thick, deeper layer of skin—is composed of collagen and elastin fibers and an extracellular matrix, which contributes to skin's strength and pliability. Collagen fibers give skin its strength, and elastin fibers provide elasticity. The meshing of

---

Memory jogger

To remember the five layers of the epidermis, think, "Cozy Layers Generate Skin Barriers." In other words, the epidermis consists of the strata:

Corneum

Lucidum

Granulosum

Spinosum

Basale.

collagen and elastin determines the skin's physical characteristics. (See *Structural supports: Collagen and elastin.*)

In addition, the dermis contains:

• blood vessels and lymphatic vessels, which transport oxygen and nutrients to cells and remove waste products

• nerve fibers and hair follicles, which contribute to skin sensation, temperature regulation, and excretion and absorption through the skin

• fibroblast cells, which are important in the production of collagen and elastin.

Laying it on thick

The dermis is composed of two layers of connective tissue:

The *papillary dermis*, the outermost layer, is composed of collagen and reticular fibers, which are important in healing wounds. Capillaries in the papillary dermis carry the nourishment needed for metabolic activity.

Structural supports: Collagen and elastin

Normally, skin returns to its original position after it's pulled on. This is because of the actions of the connective tissues collagen and elastin—two key components of skin.

Understanding the components
Collagen and elastin work together to support the dermis and give skin its physical characteristics.

Collagen
Collagen fibers form tightly woven networks in the papillary layer of the dermis, or thick bundles paralleling the skin's surface. These fibers are relatively inextensible and nonelastic and, therefore, give the dermis high tensile strength. In addition, collagen constitutes approximately 70% of the skin's dry weight and is the skin's principal structural body protein.

Elastin
Elastin is made up of wavy fibers that intertwine with collagen in horizontal arrangements at the lower dermis and vertical arrangements at the epidermal margin. Elastin makes skin pliable and is the structural protein that enables extensibility in the dermis.

Seeing the effects of age
As a person ages, collagen and elastin fibers break down and the fine lines and wrinkles that are associated with aging develop. Extensive exposure to sunlight accelerates this breakdown process. Deep wrinkles are caused by changes in facial muscles. Over time, laughing, crying, smiling, and frowning cause facial muscles to thicken and eventually cause wrinkles in the overlying skin.

Don't let your laugh lines give you worry warts. Breakdown of collagen and elastin fibers is a normal part of aging.

The *reticular dermis* is the innermost layer. It's formed by thick networks of collagen bundles that anchor it to the subcutaneous tissue and underlying supporting structures, such as fasciae, muscle, and bone.

Sebaceous glands and sweat glands

Although sebaceous glands and sweat glands appear to originate in the dermis, they're actually appendages of the epidermis that extend downward into the dermis.

Give the glands a hand!

Sebaceous glands, found primarily in the skin of the scalp, face, upper body, and genital region, are part of the same structure that contains hair follicles. These saclike glands produce sebum, a fatty substance that lubricates and softens the skin.

Don't sweat it

Sweat glands are tightly coiled tubular glands; the average person has roughly 2.6 million of them. They're present throughout the body in varying amounts: the palms and soles have many but the external ear, lip margins, nail beds, and glans penis have none.

The secreting portion of the sweat gland originates in the dermis and the outlet is on the surface of the skin. The sympathetic nervous system regulates the production of sweat, which, in turn, helps control body temperature.

There are two types of sweat glands:

Eccrine glands are active at birth and are found throughout the body. They're most dense on the palms, soles of the feet, and forehead. These glands connect to the skin's surface through pores and produce sweat that lacks proteins and fatty acids. Eccrine glands are smaller than apocrine glands.

Apocrine glands begin to function at puberty. These glands open into hair follicles; therefore, most are found in areas where hair typically grows, such as the scalp, groin, and axillary region. The coiled secreting portion of the gland lies deep in the dermis (deeper than eccrine glands), and a duct connects it to the upper portion of the hair follicle. The sweat produced by apocrine glands contains water, sodium, chloride, proteins, and fatty acids. It's thicker than the sweat produced by eccrine glands and has a milky-white or yellowish tinge. (See *Oh no, B.O.!* page 6.)

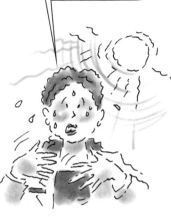

The sympathetic nervous system regulates the production of sweat. This actually helps keep the body cool on hot days.

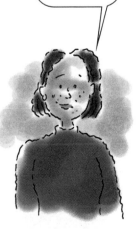

Apocrine sweat glands begin to function at puberty. Lucky me!

Oh no, B.O.!

The sweat produced by apocrine glands contains the same water, sodium, and chloride found in the sweat produced by eccrine glands. However, it also contains proteins and fatty acids. The unpleasant odor associated with sweat comes from the interaction of bacteria with these proteins and fatty acids.

Subcutaneous tissue

Subcutaneous tissue, or hypodermis, is a subdermal (below the skin) layer of loose connective tissue that contains major blood vessels, lymph vessels, and nerves. Subcutaneous tissue:
• has a high proportion of fat cells and contains fewer small blood vessels than the dermis
• varies in thickness depending on body type and location
• constitutes 15% to 20% of a man's weight; 20% to 25% of a woman's weight
• insulates the body
• absorbs shocks to the skeletal system
• helps skin move easily over underlying structures.

Blood supply

The skin receives its blood supply through vessels that originate in the underlying muscle tissue. Here, arteries branch into smaller vessels, which then branch into the network of capillaries that permeate the dermis and subcutaneous tissue.

The thin and thinner of it

Within the vascular system, only capillaries have walls thin enough (typically only a single layer of endothelial cells) to let solutes pass through. These thin walls allow nutrients and oxygen to pass from the bloodstream into the interstitial space around skin cells. At the same time, waste products pass into the capillaries and are carried away. The pressure of arterial blood entering the capillaries is approximately 30 mm Hg. The pressure of venous blood leaving the capillaries is approximately 10 mm Hg. This 20–mm Hg difference in pressure within the capillaries is quite low when compared with the pressure found in the larger arteries in the body (85 to 100 mm Hg), which is known as *blood pressure.* (See *Fluid movement through capillaries.*)

Now I get it!

Fluid movement through capillaries

The movement of fluids through capillaries—a process called *capillary filtration*—results from blood pushing against the walls of the capillary. That pressure, called *hydrostatic* or *fluid-pushing pressure,* forces fluids and solutes through the capillary wall.

When the hydrostatic pressure inside a capillary is greater than the pressure in the surrounding interstitial space, fluids and solutes inside the capillary are forced out into the interstitial space, as shown here. When the pressure inside the capillary is less than the pressure outside, fluids and solutes move back into it.

Solutes

Fluids and solutes move out of the capillary.

Hydrostatic pressure

Capillary

Capillary wall

Lymphatic system

The skin's lymphatic system helps remove waste products from the dermis.

Go with the flow

Lymphatic vessels, or *lymphatics* for short, are similar to capillaries in that they're thin-walled, permeable vessels. However, lymphatics aren't part of the blood circulatory system. Instead, the lymphatics belong to a separate system that removes proteins, large waste products, and excess fluids from the interstitial spaces in skin and then transports them to the venous circulation. The lymphatics merge into two main trunks—the thoracic duct and the right lymphatic duct—which empty into the junction of the subclavian and internal jugular veins.

Functions of the skin

Skin performs, or participates in, a host of vital functions, including:

- protection of internal structures
- sensory perception
- thermoregulation
- excretion
- metabolism
- absorption
- social communication.

  Damage to skin impairs its ability to carry out these important functions. Let's take a closer look at each.

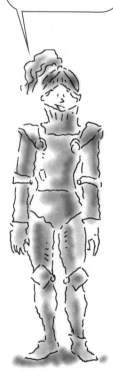

Sometimes you need more protection than at other times. Skin acts as a physical barrier to such invaders as microorganisms.

Protection

Skin acts as a physical barrier to microorganisms and foreign matter, protecting the body against infection. It also protects underlying tissue and structures from mechanical injury. Consider the feet for a moment. As a person walks or runs, the soles of the feet withstand a tremendous amount of force, yet the underlying tissue and bone structures remain unharmed. Finally, skin helps maintain a stable environment inside the body by preventing the loss of water, electrolytes, proteins, and other substances. Any damage — any wound — jeopardizes this protection. However, when damaged, skin goes into repair mode to restore full protection by stepping up the normal process of cell replacement.

Sensory perception

Nerve endings in the skin allow a person to literally touch the world around him. Sensory nerve fibers originate in the nerve roots along the spine and supply specific areas of the skin known as dermatomes. Dermatomes are used to document sensory function. This same network helps a person avoid injury by making him aware of pain, pressure, heat, and cold.

Just sensational

Sensory nerves exist throughout the skin; however, some areas are more sensitive than others — for example, the fingertips are more sensitive than the back. Sensation allows us to identify potential dangers and avoid injury. Any loss or reduction of sensation, local or general, increases the chance of injury.

Thermoregulation

Thermoregulation, or control of body temperature, involves the concerted effort of nerves, blood vessels, and eccrine glands in the dermis.

Warming up

When skin is exposed to cold or internal body temperature falls, blood vessels constrict, reducing blood flow and thereby conserving body heat.

Cooling down

Similarly, if skin becomes too hot or internal body temperature rises, small arteries within the skin dilate, increasing the blood flow, and sweat production increases to promote cooling.

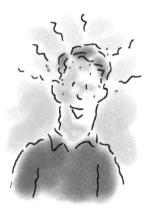

Excretion

Unlikely as it may seem at first, the skin is an excretory organ. Excretion through the skin plays an important role in thermoregulation, electrolyte balance, and hydration. In addition, sebum excretion helps maintain the skin's integrity and suppleness.

Water works

Through its more than two million pores, skin efficiently transmits trace amounts of water and body wastes to the environment. At the same time, it prevents dehydration by ensuring that the body doesn't lose too much water. Sweat carries water and salt to the skin surface, where it evaporates, aiding thermoregulation and electrolyte balance. In addition, a small amount of water evaporates directly from the skin itself each day. A normal adult loses about 500 ml of water per day this way. While the skin is busy regulating fluids that are leaving the body, it's equally busy preventing unwanted or dangerous fluids from entering the body.

Metabolism

Skin also helps to maintain the mineralization of bones and teeth.

Let the sun shine in

A photochemical reaction in the skin produces vitamin D, which is crucial to the metabolism of calcium and phosphate. These minerals, in turn, play a central role in the health of bones and teeth. When skin is exposed to sunlight—the UV spectrum in sunlight, to be specific—vitamin D is synthesized in a photochemical reaction. Keep in mind, however, that although some sunlight works wonders, overexposure to UV light causes skin damage that reduces its ability to function properly.

Absorption

Some drugs (and, unfortunately, some toxic substances — pesticides, for example) can be absorbed directly through the skin and into the bloodstream. This process has been used to treat certain disorders via skin patch drug delivery systems. One of the best-known examples of this is "the patch" used in some nicotine withdrawal programs. However, today this technology is also used to administer some forms of hormone replacement therapy, nitroglycerin, and some pain medications.

Social communication

A commonly overlooked but important function of the skin is its role in self-esteem development and social communication. Every time a person looks in the mirror he decides whether he likes what he sees. Although bone structure, body type, teeth, and hair (or lack thereof!) all have an impact, the condition and characteristics of skin can have the greatest impact on a person's self-esteem. Ask any teenager with acne. If a person likes what he sees, self-esteem rises; if he doesn't, it sags.

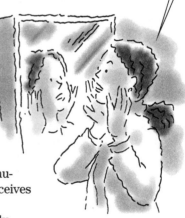

Unfortunately, in some cases, social communication is only skin deep. Good skin can lead to increased self-esteem.

What you see

Virtually every interpersonal exchange includes the non-verbal languages of facial expression and body posture. Level of self-esteem and skin characteristics — which are visible at all times — have an impact on how a person communicates, both verbally and nonverbally, and how a listener receives the person communicating.

Because the physical characteristics of skin are so closely linked to self-perception, there has been a proliferation of skin care products and surgical techniques offered to keep skin looking young and healthy.

Aging and skin function

Over time, skin loses its ability to function as efficiently or as effectively as it once did. (See *How skin ages*.) As a result, the golden years of life place a person at greater risk for such injuries as pressure ulcers and tumors as well as various other skin conditions.

How skin ages

This table lists skin changes that normally occur with aging.

Change	Findings in elderly people
Pigmentation	• Pale color
Thickness	• Wrinkling, especially on the face, arms, and legs • Parchmentlike appearance, especially over bony prominences and on the dorsal surfaces of the hands, feet, arms, and legs
Moisture	• Dry, flaky, and rough
Turgor	• "Tents" and stands alone
Texture	• Numerous creases and lines

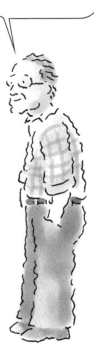

As a person ages, the skin undergoes many changes that can increase the risk of wounds.

What's ahead

Although the entire body changes a great deal over time, several important changes in the skin increase the risk of wounds as a person ages. These include:
• a 50% reduction in the cell turnover rate in the stratum corneum (outermost layer) and a 20% reduction in dermal thickness
• generalized reduction in dermal vascularization and an associated drop in blood flow to the skin
• redistribution of subcutaneous tissue, which contains fewer fat cells in older people, to the stomach and thighs
• flattening of papillae in the dermoepidermal junction (meeting of the epidermis and dermis), which reduces adhesion between layers
• a drop in the number of Langerhans' cells (immune macrophages that attack invading germs) present in the skin
• a 50% decline in the number of fibroblasts and mast cells (cells that play a key role in the inflammatory response)
• marked reduction in the ability to sense pressure, heat, and cold, even though the same number of nerve endings in the skin are retained
• a significant decline in the number of sweat glands
• poorer absorption through the skin
• a reduction in the skin's ability to synthesize vitamin D.

What it means

As a person ages, physiologic changes increase the risk of various injuries. For example, older adults:

• bruise easier and are more prone to edema around wounds due to reduced skin vascularization

• are more likely to suffer pressure and thermal (hot and cold) damage to the skin due to diminished sensation

• have a higher incidence of ischemia (cell damage resulting from too little oxygen reaching cells) in compressed tissue because bony areas have less subcutaneous cushioning and decreased sensation causes an elderly person to be less sensitive to the discomfort of remaining in one position for too long

• risk hyperthermia and hypothermia because of decreased subcutaneous tissue

• have fewer sweat glands and, therefore, produce less sweat, which hinders thermoregulation and increases the risk of hyperthermia

• have a higher risk of infection because thinner skin is a less effective barrier to germs and allergens and because the skin contains fewer Langerhans' cells to fight infection and fewer mast cells to mediate the inflammatory response

• are slower to exhibit a sensitization response (redness, heat, discomfort) due to the reduction in Langerhans' cells, resulting in overuse of topical medications and more severe allergic reactions (because signs aren't evident early on)

• risk overdose of transdermal medications when poor absorption prompts them to reapply the medication too often

• have a much higher incidence of shear and tear injuries due to compromised skin layer adhesion and less flexible collagen

• have a reduction in sensation that prevents them from noticing the discomfort associated with impending skin tears.

A look at wounds

Any break in the skin is considered a wound. Wounds can result from a planned event, such as surgery, or from an unexpected event, such as an accident, trauma, or exposure to pressure, heat, sun, or chemicals. Tissue damage in wounds varies widely, from a superficial break in the epithelium to deep trauma that involves the muscle and bone. A "clean" wound is a wound produced by surgery. A wound is described as "dirty" if it may contain bacteria or debris. Trauma typically produces dirty wounds. The rate of recovery is influenced by

Oh no! Trauma can cause some pretty dirty wounds.

the extent and type of damage incurred as well as other intrinsic factors, such as patient circulation, nutrition, and hydration. However, regardless of the cause of a wound, the healing process is much the same in all cases.

Types of wound healing

Wounds are classified by the way the wound closes. A wound can close by primary intention, secondary intention, or tertiary intention.

Primary intention

Primary healing involves reepithelialization, in which the skin's outer layer grows closed. Cells grow in from the margins of the wound and out from epithelial cells lining the hair follicles and sweat glands.

Just a scratch

Wounds that heal through primary intention are, most commonly, superficial wounds that involve only the epidermis and don't involve the loss of tissue — a first-degree burn, for example. However, a wound that has well-approximated edges (edges that can be pulled together to meet neatly), such as a surgical incision, also heals through primary intention. Because there's no loss of tissue and little risk of infection, the healing process is predictable. These wounds usually heal in 4 to 14 days and result in minimal scarring.

Secondary intention

A wound that involves some degree of tissue loss heals by secondary intention. The edges of these wounds can't be easily approximated, and the wound itself is described as partial thickness or full thickness, depending on its depth:
• Partial-thickness wounds extend through the epidermis and into, but not through, the dermis.
• Full-thickness wounds extend through the epidermis and dermis and may involve subcutaneous tissue, muscle and, possibly, bone.

It's important to reposition patients on bed rest often to avoid pressure ulcers — one type of wound that heals by secondary intention.

Getting under the skin

During healing, wounds that heal by secondary intention fill with granulation tissue, a scar forms, and reepithelialization occurs, primarily from the wound edges. Pressure ulcers, burns, dehisced surgical wounds, and traumatic injuries are examples of this type of wound. These wounds also take longer to heal, result in scarring, and have a higher rate of complications than wounds that heal by primary intention.

⚝ Tertiary intention

When a wound is intentionally kept open to allow edema or infection to resolve or to permit removal of exudate, the wound heals by tertiary intention, or delayed primary intention. These wounds result in more scarring than wounds that heal by primary intention but less than wounds that heal by secondary intention.

Phases of wound healing

The healing process is the same for all wounds, whether the cause is mechanical, chemical, or thermal.

Don't let it phase you

Health care professionals discuss the process of wound healing in four specific phases:
- hemostasis
- inflammation
- proliferation
- maturation.

　　Although this categorization is useful, it's important to remember that healing rarely occurs in this strict order. Typically, the phases of wound healing overlap. (See *How wounds heal.*)

Hemostasis

Immediately after an injury, the body releases chemical mediators and intercellular messengers called growth factors that begin the process of cleaning and healing the wound.

Slow that flow!

When blood vessels are damaged, the small muscles in the walls of the vessels contract (vasoconstriction), reducing the flow of blood to the injury and minimizing blood loss. Vasoconstriction can last as long as 30 minutes.

　　Next, blood leaking from the inflamed, dilated, or broken vessels begins to coagulate. Collagen fibers in the wall of the damaged blood vessels activate the platelets in the blood in the wound. Aided by the action of prostaglandins, the platelets enlarge and stick together to form a temporary plug in the blood vessel, which helps prevent further bleeding. The platelets also release additional vasoconstrictors — such as serotonin — which help to prevent further blood loss. Thrombin forms in a cascade of events stimulated by the platelets, and a clot forms to close the small vessels and stop bleeding.

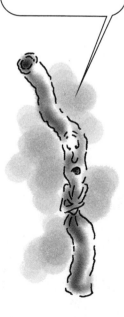

Vasoconstriction reduces the flow of blood to the injury, which minimizes blood loss and therefore promotes hemostasis.

Now I get it!

How wounds heal

The healing process begins at the instant of injury and proceeds through a repair "cascade," as outlined here.

1. When tissue is damaged, serotonin, histamine, prostaglandins, and blood from the injured vessels fill the area. Blood platelets form a clot, and fibrin in the clot binds the wound edges together.

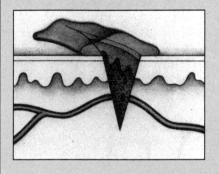

2. Lymphocytes initiate the inflammatory response, increasing capillary permeability. Wound edges swell; white blood cells from surrounding vessels move in and ingest bacteria and cellular debris, demolishing the clot. Redness, warmth, swelling, pain, and loss of function may occur.

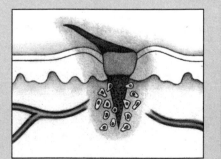

3. Adjacent healthy tissue supplies blood, nutrients, fibroblasts, proteins, and other building materials needed to form soft, pink, and highly vascular granulation tissue, which begins to bridge the area. Inflammation may decrease, or signs and symptoms of infection (increased swelling, increased pain, fever, and pus-filled discharge) may develop.

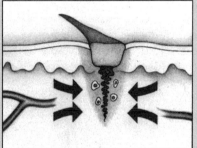

4. Fibroblasts in the granulation tissue secrete collagen, a gluelike substance. Collagen fibers crisscross the area, forming scar tissue.

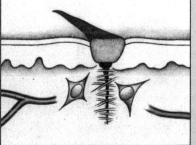

5. Meanwhile, epithelial cells at the wound edge multiply and migrate toward the wound center. A new layer of surface cells replaces the layer that was destroyed. New, healthy tissue or granulation tissue (if the blood supply is inadequate) appears.

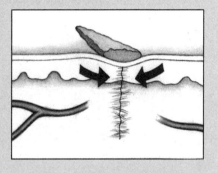

6. Damaged tissue (including lymphatics, blood vessels, and stromal matrices) regenerates. Collagen fibers shorten, and the scar diminishes in size. Scar size may decrease and normal function return or the scar may hypertrophy, leading to the formation of a keloid and the development of contractures.

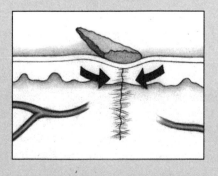

This initial phase of wound healing occurs almost immediately after the injury occurs and works quickly (within minutes) in small wounds. It's less effective in stopping the bleeding in larger wounds.

Inflammation

The inflammatory phase is both a defense mechanism and a crucial component of the healing process. (See *Understanding the inflammatory response.*) During this phase, the wound is cleaned and the process of rebuilding begins. This phase is marked by swelling, redness, and heat at the wound site.

During the inflammatory phase, vascular permeability increases, permitting serous fluid carrying small amounts of cell and plasma protein to accumulate in the tissue around the wound (edema). The accumulation of fluid causes the damaged tissue to appear swollen, red, and warm to the touch.

> Way to go! Neutrophils infiltrate the wound in order to remove or destroy bacteria and other contaminants through a process called phagocytosis.

Seek and destroy

During the early phase of the inflammatory process, neutrophils (one type of white blood cell) enter the wound. The primary role of neutrophils is phagocytosis,

---

Now I get it!

Understanding the inflammatory response

The flowchart below outlines the sequence of events in the inflammatory process.

Microorganisms invade damaged tissue.

⬇

Basophils release heparin, and histamine and kinin production occurs.

⬇

Vasodilation occurs along with increased capillary permeability.

⬇

Blood flow increases to the affected tissues and fluid collects within them.

⬇

Neutrophils flock to the invasion site to engulf and destroy microorganisms from dying cells.

⬇

This repairs the tissue.

or the removal and destruction of bacteria and other contaminants.

As neutrophil infiltration slows, monocytes appear. Monocytes are converted into activated macrophages and continue the job of cleaning the wound. The macrophages play a key role early in the process of granulation and reepithelialization by producing growth factors and by attracting the cells needed for the formation of new blood vessels and collagen.

Telling time

The inflammatory phase of healing is important for preventing wound infection. The process is negatively influenced if the patient has a systemic condition that suppresses his immune system or if he's undergoing immunosuppressive therapy. In clean wounds, the inflammatory response lasts about 36 hours. In dirty or infected wounds, the response can last much longer.

Proliferation

During the proliferation phase of the healing process, the body:
- fills the wound with connective tissue (granulation)
- contracts the wound edges (contraction)
- covers the wound with epithelium (epithelialization).

Presto change-o!

All wounds go through the proliferation phase, but it takes much longer in wounds with extensive tissue loss. Although phases overlap, wound granulation generally starts when the inflammatory response is complete. As the inflammatory phase subsides, the wound exudate (drainage) begins to decrease.

The proliferation phase involves regeneration of blood vessels (angiogenesis) and the formation of connective or granulation tissue. The development of granulation tissue requires an adequate supply of blood and nutrients. Endothelial cells in blood vessels in surrounding tissue reconstruct damaged or destroyed vessels by first migrating and then proliferating to form new capillary beds. As the beds form, this area of the wound takes on a red, granular appearance. This tissue is a good defense against contaminants, but it's also quite fragile and bleeds easily.

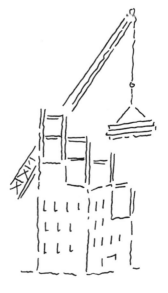

The rebuilding process

During the proliferation phase, growth factors prompt fibroblasts to migrate to the wound. Fibroblasts are the most common cell in connective tissue; they're responsible for making fibers and ground substance, also known as extracellular matrix, which provides support to cells. At first, fibroblasts populate just the margins of the wound; they later spread over the entire wound surface.

Fibroblasts have the important task of synthesizing collagen fibers which, in turn, produce keratinocyte, a growth factor needed for reepithelialization. This process necessitates a delicate balance of collagen synthesis and lysis (making new and removing old). If the process yields too much collagen, increased scarring results. If the process yields too little collagen, scar tissue is weak and easily ruptured. Because fibroblasts require a supply of oxygen to perform their important role, capillary bed regeneration is crucial to the process.

Fibroblasts may be small but we have a big job. We synthesize collagen, which is necessary for proper wound healing.

Pulling it all together

As healing progresses, myofibroblasts and the newly formed collagen fibers contract, pulling the wound edges toward each other. Contraction reduces the amount of granulation tissue needed to fill the wound, thereby speeding the healing process. (See *Contraction vs. contracture.*)

Complete healing occurs only after epithelial cells have completely covered the surface of the wound. As this occurs, keratinocytes switch from a migratory mode to a differentiative mode. The epidermis thickens and becomes differentiated, and the wound is closed. Any remaining scab comes off and the new epidermis is toughened by the production of keratin, which also returns the skin to its original color.

Now I get it!

Contraction vs. contracture

Contraction and contracture occur during the wound healing process. While they have mechanisms in common, it's important to understand how contraction and contracture differ:
• Contraction, a desirable process that occurs during healing, is the process by which the edges of a wound pull toward the center of the wound to close it. Contraction continues to close the wound until tension in the surrounding skin causes it to slow and then stop.
• Contracture is an undesirable process and a common complication of burn scarring. Typically, contracture occurs after healing is complete. Contracture involves an inordinate amount of pulling or shortening of tissue, resulting in an area of tissue with only limited ability to move. It's especially problematic over joints, which may be pulled to a flexed position. Stretching is the only way to overcome contracture, and patients typically require physical therapy.

Maturation

The final phase of wound healing is maturation, which is marked by the shrinking and strengthening of the scar. This is a gradual, transitional phase of healing that can continue for months or even years after the wound has closed.

During this phase, fibroblasts leave the site of the wound, vascularization is reduced, the scar shrinks and becomes pale, and the mature scar forms. If the wound involved extensive tissue destruction, the scar won't contain hair, sweat, or sebaceous glands.

The wound gradually gains tensile strength. In primary intention wounds, tissues will achieve approximately 30% to 50% of their original strength between days 1 and 14. When fully healed, tissue will achieve, at best, approximately 80% of its original strength. Scar tissue will always be less elastic than the surrounding skin.

Factors that affect healing

The healing process is affected by many factors. The most important influences include:

- nutrition
- oxygenation
- infection
- age
- chronic health conditions
- medications
- smoking.

Nutrition

Proper nutrition is arguably the most important factor affecting wound healing. Unfortunately, malnutrition is a common finding among patients with wounds; it's reported in 30% of adult surgical patients and 45% to 57% of nonsurgical patients. For older adults, the problem is more pervasive. Malnutrition is reported in 53% to 74% of older hospitalized patients.

Poor nutrition prolongs hospitalization and increases the risk of medical complications, with the severity of complications being directly related to the severity of the malnutrition. In older patients, malnutrition is known to increase the risk of pressure ulcers and delay wound healing. It may also contribute to poor tensile strength in healing wounds, with an associated increase in the risk of wound dehiscence. (See *Tips for detecting nutritional problems*, page 20.)

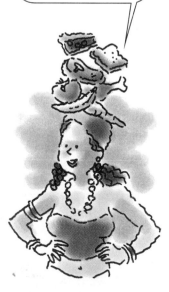

Because nutrition plays a critical role in wound healing, you need to make sure that your patient eats a balanced diet.

Tips for detecting nutritional problems

Nutritional problems may stem from physical conditions, drugs, diet, or lifestyle factors. The list below can help you identify risk factors that make your patient particularly susceptible to nutritional problems.

Physical condition
- Chronic illnesses such as diabetes and neurologic, cardiac, or thyroid problems
- Family history of diabetes or heart disease
- Draining wounds or fistulas
- Weight issues—weight loss of 5% of normal body weight; weight less than 90% of ideal body weight; weight gain or loss of 10 lb or more in last 6 months; obesity; or weight gain of 20% above normal body weight
- History of GI disturbances
- Anorexia or bulimia
- Depression or anxiety
- Severe trauma
- Recent chemotherapy or radiation therapy
- Physical limitations, such as paresis or paralysis

- Recent major surgery
- Pregnancy, especially teen or multiple-birth pregnancy

Drugs and diet
- Fad diets
- Steroid, diuretic, or antacid use
- Mouth, tooth, or denture problems
- Excessive alcohol intake
- Strict vegetarian diet
- Liquid diet or nothing by mouth for more than 3 days

Lifestyle factors
- Lack of support from family or friends
- Financial problems

Protein is key...

Protein is critical for wounds to heal properly. In fact, a person needs to double the recommended dietary allowance of protein (from 0.8 g/kg/day to 1.6 g/kg/day) before tissue even begins to heal. If a significant amount of body weight has been lost in connection with the injury, as much as 50% of the lost weight must be regained before healing will begin. A patient who lacks protein reserves heals slowly, if at all, and a patient who's borderline malnourished can easily become malnourished under this demand.

The body needs protein to form collagen during the proliferation phase. Without adequate protein, collagen formation is reduced or delayed and the healing process slows. Studies of malnourished patients indicate that they have lower levels of serum albumin, which results in slower oxygen diffusion and, in turn, a reduction in the ability of neutrophils to kill bacteria. Wound exudate alone can contain up to 100 g of protein per day.

Protein is a critical component of wound healing. Double up on your patient's protein intake to ensure proper and timely healing.

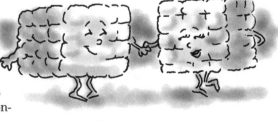

...but other nutrients are also necessary

Fatty acids (lipids) are used in cell structures and play a role in the inflammatory process. Also, vitamins C, B-complex, A, and E and the minerals iron, copper, zinc, and calcium are important in the healing process. A zinc deficiency adversely affects the proliferation phase by slowing the rate of epithelialization and decreasing the strength of collagen produced—and, thus, the strength of the wound.

In addition to protein and zinc, collagen synthesis requires supplies of carbohydrates and fat. Collagen cross-linking requires adequate amounts of vitamins A and C, iron, and copper. Vitamin C, iron, and zinc are important to developing tensile strength during the maturation phase of wound healing.

Oxygenation

Healing depends on a regular supply of oxygen. For example, oxygen is critical for leukocytes to destroy bacteria and for fibroblasts to stimulate collagen synthesis. If the supply is hindered by poor blood flow to the area of the wound or if the patient's ability to take in adequate oxygen is impaired, the result is the same—impaired healing.

Possible causes of inadequate blood flow to the area of the wound include pressure, arterial occlusion, or prolonged vasoconstriction, possibly associated with such medical conditions as peripheral vascular disease and atherosclerosis. Possible causes of a lower than necessary systemic blood oxygenation include:
- inadequate oxygen intake
- hypothermia or hyperthermia
- anemia
- alkalemia
- other medical conditions such as chronic obstructive pulmonary disease.

Infection

Infection can be systemic or localized in the wound. A systemic infection, such as pneumonia or tuberculosis, increases the patient's metabolism and thus consumes the fluids, nutrients, and oxygen the body needs for healing.

A localized infection in the wound itself is more common. Remember, any break in the skin allows bacteria to enter. The infection may occur as part of the injury or may develop later in the healing process. For example, when the inflammatory phase lingers, wound healing is delayed and metabolic by-products of bacterial ingestion accumulate in the wound. This buildup interferes with the formation of new blood vessels and the synthesis of collagen. Infection can also occur in a wound that has been healing normally. This is especially true for larger wounds involving extensive tissue damage. New or increased pain, redness, heat,

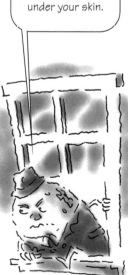

Pay no attention to me! I'm just looking for a way to get under your skin.

and drainage are signs of a new infection. In any case, healing can't progress until the cause of infection is addressed.

In patients in long-term care facilities, infection may result from fecal contamination. Fecal incontinence affects 20% of long-term care patients and is associated with increased mortality. Typically, those affected are patients with poorer overall health.

Age

Skin changes that occur with aging cause healing time to be prolonged in elderly patients. Although delayed healing is partially due to physiologic changes, it's usually complicated by other problems associated with aging, such as poor nutrition and hydration, the presence of a chronic condition, or the use of multiple medications. (See *Effects of aging on wound healing.*)

Chronic health conditions

Respiratory problems, atherosclerosis, diabetes, and malignancies can increase the risk of wounds and interfere with wound healing. These conditions can interfere with systemic and peripheral oxygenation and nutrition, which affect healing.

Getting complicated

Impaired circulation, a common problem for patients with diabetes and other disorders, can cause tissue hypoxia (lack of oxygen). Neuropathy associated with diabetes reduces a per-

(Text continues on page 23.)

> Don't forget that such health problems as respiratory disorders, atherosclerosis, diabetes, and malignancies not only increase the risk of wounds but also hinder healing.

Effects of aging on wound healing

In older adults, the following factors impede wound healing:
• slower turnover rate in epidermal cells
• poorer oxygenation at the wound due to increasingly fragile capillaries and a reduction in skin vascularization
• altered nutrition and fluid intake resulting from physical changes that can accompany aging, such as reduced saliva production, a declining sense of smell and taste, or decreased stomach motility
• altered nutrition and fluid intake attributable to troubling personal or social issues, such as loose-fitting dentures, financial concerns, eating alone after the death of a spouse, or problems preparing or obtaining food
• impaired function of the respiratory or immune systems
• reduced dermal and subcutaneous mass leading to an increased risk of chronic pressure ulcers
• healed wounds that lack tensile strength and are prone to reinjury.

A close look at skin layers

Skin is made up of separate layers that function as a single unit. Two distinct layers of skin, the epidermis and dermis, lie above a layer of subcutaneous fatty tissue (sometimes called the *hypodermis*).

It's more than skin deep. The integument protects inner body structures, perceives touch, regulates body temperature, and excretes certain body fluids.

Epidermis

Dermal papillae

Dermis

Subcutaneous tissue

Vein

Artery

Stratum corneum

Stratum granulosum

Stratum spinosum

Stratum basale

Free nerve ending

Meissner's corpuscle

Sebaceous gland

Pore of sweat gland

Arrector pili muscle

Krause's end-bulb

Collagen fiber

Ruffini's corpuscle

Hair bulb

Sensory nerve fibers

Eccrine sweat gland

Autonomic nerve fibers

Subcutaneous fatty tissue

Wound color cues

Wound color can guide your specific management approach and tell you how well a wound is healing. The Red-Yellow-Black Classification System is a commonly used approach that can help simplify your assessment. Remember, if you note more than one color in a wound, classify the wound according to the least healthy color.

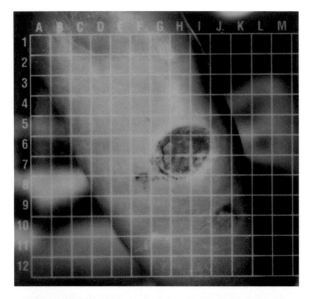

Red wounds

Red, the color of healthy granulation tissue, indicates normal healing. When a wound begins to heal, a layer of pale pink granulation tissue covers the wound bed. As this layer thickens, it becomes beefy red. This photo shows a diabetic foot ulcer with a granulation tissue base.

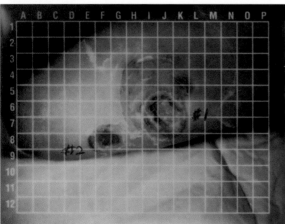

Yellow wounds

Yellow slough or dead tissue on the wound base is usually fibrin left over from the healing process. This slough, or soft necrotic tissue, is a medium for bacteria growth. This photo shows a diabetic foot ulcer with a slough-covered base and calloused edges.

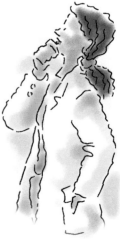

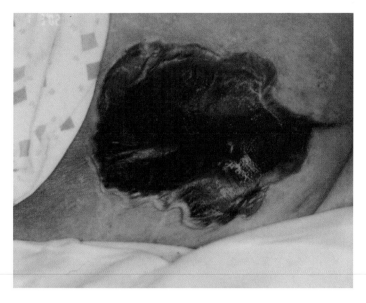

Black wounds

Black, the least healthy wound color, signals necrosis. Dead avascular tissue slows healing and provides a site for microorganisms to proliferate. The photo at left shows a black pressure ulcer; the one below it shows black ischemic toe ulcers.

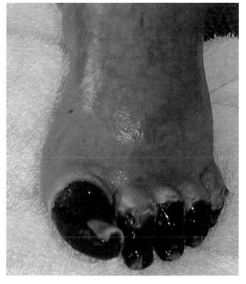

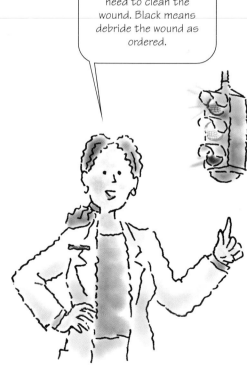

Detecting wound dehiscence

Although surgical wounds typically heal without incident, occasionally the edges of a wound may fail to join or may separate after they begin to heal. This development, called *wound dehiscence,* may lead to evisceration, an even more serious complication, in which a portion of a viscus (in an abdominal incision, usually a bowel loop) protrudes through the incision. These photos illustrate a dehisced abdominal wound and a healing dehisced abdominal wound.

Dehisced abdominal wound (with a colostomy)

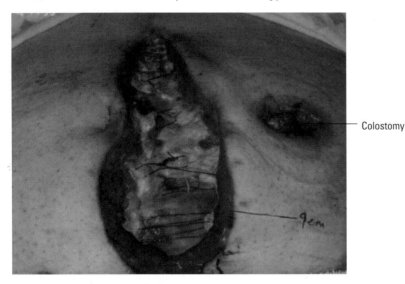

— Colostomy

Dehisced healing abdominal incision

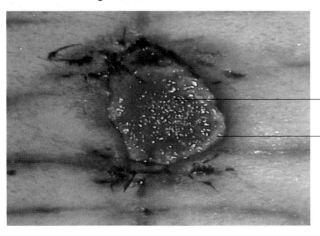

— Red granulation tissue

— Yellow fibrin slough

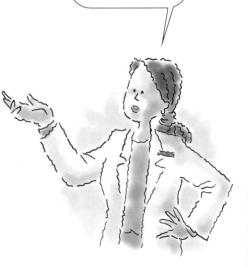

Note the red granulation tissue in the center and the yellow fibrin slough at the wound bed edges.

son's ability to sense pressure. As a result, a diabetic patient may experience trauma, especially to the feet, without realizing it. Insulin dependency can impair leukocyte function, which adversely affects cell proliferation.

Hemiplegia and quadriplegia involve the breakdown of muscle tissue and reduction in the padding around the large bones of the lower body. Because a patient with one of these conditions lacks sensation, he's at risk for developing chronic pressure ulcers.

Night and day shifts

Normally, a healthy person shifts position every 15 minutes or so, even during sleep. This prevents tissue damage due to ischemia. Anything that impairs the ability to sense pressure, including the use of pain medications, spinal cord lesions, or cognitive impairment, puts the patient at risk (the patient can't feel the growing discomfort of pressure and respond to it).

Other conditions that can delay healing include dehydration, end-stage renal disease, thyroid disease, heart failure, peripheral vascular disease, and vasculitis and other collagen vascular disorders.

Medications

Any medication that reduces a patient's movement, circulation, or metabolic function, such as sedatives and tranquilizers, has the potential to inhibit the patient's ability to sense and respond to pressure. Also, because movement promotes adequate oxygenation, lack of motion means that peripheral blood delivers less oxygen to the extremities than it should. This is especially problematic for older adults. Remember, oxygen is important; without it, the healing process slows and the potential for complications rises.

Some medications, such as steroids and chemotherapeutic agents, reduce the body's ability to mount an appropriate inflammatory response. This interrupts the inflammatory phase of healing and can dramatically lengthen healing time, especially in patients with compromised immune systems such as those with acquired immunodeficiency syndrome.

Medications, particularly sedatives, can also cause complications.

Smoking

Carbon monoxide, a component of cigarette smoke, binds to the hemoglobin in blood in the place of oxygen. This significantly reduces the amount of oxygen circulating in the bloodstream, which can impede wound healing. To some extent, this reaction also occurs in people regularly exposed to second-hand smoke.

Complications of wound healing

The most common complications associated with wound healing are hemorrhage, dehiscence and evisceration, infection, and fistula formation.

Hemorrhage

Internal hemorrhage (bleeding) can result in the formation of a hematoma—a blood clot that solidifies to form a hard lump under the skin. Hematomas are commonly found around bruises.

External hemorrhage is visible bleeding from the wound. External bleeding during healing isn't unusual because the newly developed blood vessels are fragile and rupture easily. This is one reason a wound needs to be protected by a dressing. However, each time the new blood vessels suffer damage, healing is delayed while repairs are made.

Dehiscence and evisceration

Dehiscence is a separation of skin and tissue layers. It's most likely to occur 3 to 11 days after the injury was sustained and may follow surgery. Evisceration is similar but involves protrusion of underlying visceral organs as well. (See *Recognizing dehiscence and evisceration*.)

Dehiscence and evisceration may constitute a surgical emergency, especially if they involve an abdominal wound. If a wound opens without evisceration, it may need to heal by secondary intention. Poor nutrition and advanced age are two factors that increase a patient's risk of dehiscence and evisceration.

Infection

Infection is a relatively common complication of wound healing that should be addressed promptly. Infection can lead to a cellulitis or bacterial infection that spreads to surrounding tissue. Signs that infection may be at work include:
• redness and warmth of the margins and tissue around the wound
• fever
• edema
• pain (or a sudden increase in pain)
• pus
• increase in exudate or a change in its color
• odor
• discoloration of granulation tissue
• further wound breakdown or lack of progress toward healing.

Recognizing dehiscence and evisceration

In wound dehiscence (top), the layers of a wound separate. In evisceration (bottom), the viscera (in this case, a bowel loop) protrude through the wound.

Wound dehiscence

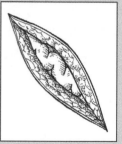

Evisceration of bowel loop

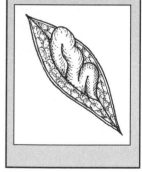

Fistula

A fistula is an abnormal passage between two organs or between an organ and the skin. In a wound, it may appear as undermining or a sinus tract in the skin around the wound. If a sinus tract (or tunneling) is present, it's important to determine its extent and direction.

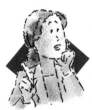

Quick quiz

1. The outermost layer of the skin is the:
   A. epidermis.
   B. dermis.
   C. hypodermis.
   D. subdermal layer.

Answer: A. The epidermis is the outermost layer of the skin. It's composed of epithelial tissue and is supported by the dermis.

2. The layer of skin that contains apocrine sweat glands is the:
   A. stratum corneum.
   B. dermis.
   C. subcutaneous tissue.
   D. stratum basale.

Answer: B. Apocrine glands are situated in the dermis and have ducts that empty into hair follicles.

3. The structures that deliver oxygen and nutrients to skin cells are:
   A. dermatomes.
   B. lymphatics.
   C. capillaries.
   D. quadratics.

Answer: C. A rich network of capillaries delivers oxygen to the skin's cells.

4. The main functions of the skin include:
   A. support, nourishment, and sensation.
   B. protection, sensory perception, and temperature regulation.
   C. fluid transport, sensory perception, and aging regulation.
   D. support, protection, and communication.

Answer: B. The skin's main functions involve protection from in-jury, noxious chemicals, and bacterial invasion; sensory percep-tion of touch, temperature, and pain; and regulation of body heat.

5.   Which type of wound closes by primary intention?
  A.   Second-degree burn
  B.   Pressure ulcer
  C.   Traumatic injury
  D.   Surgical incision

Answer: D. A surgical incision is an example of a wound that closes by primary intention, in which there's no deep tissue loss and the wound edges are well approximated.

6.   Which phase of the wound healing process is responsible for cleaning the wound and starting the rebuilding process?
  A.   Hemostasis
  B.   Inflammation
  C.   Proliferation
  D.   Maturation

Answer: B. The inflammatory phase is both a defense mecha-nism that's vital to preventing infection of the wound and a crucial component of the healing process.

Scoring

☆☆☆   If you answered all six questions correctly, congrats! You've cer-tainly got this skin topic covered!

☆☆   If you answered four or five questions correctly, good job! It's our sensory perception that you're well healed.

☆   If you answered fewer than four questions correctly, don't sweat it. This is only chapter 1!

Wound assessment and monitoring

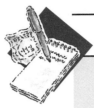

Just the facts

In this chapter, you'll learn:

♦ methods to assess the person—not just the wound

♦ ways to classify wounds according to age, depth, and color

♦ accurate documentation of wound progress

♦ tools that are available to track wound healing.

A look at wound assessment

Each time you assess a wound, remember that you're assessing a patient with a wound—not simply the wound itself. This will help keep you focused on the big picture as you perform your initial assessment and will set the stage for effective monitoring and successful healing.

Key assessment considerations

Several factors influence the body's ability to heal itself, regardless of the type of injury suffered. You should include these elements in your wound assessment:

- immune status
- blood glucose levels
- hydration
- nutrition
- blood albumin levels
- oxygen and vascular supply
- pain.

Immune status

The immune system plays a central role in wound healing. If the immune system is impaired due to such diseases as human immunodeficiency virus infection or as a result of chemotherapy or radiation, the wound should be closely monitored for impaired healing. Remember, chemotherapeutic agents aren't only used to treat cancer patients; they also may be used to treat inflammatory diseases such as arthritis. Corticosteroids may also depress immune system function.

Blood glucose levels

Blood glucose levels should be below 200 mg/dl for satisfactory healing, regardless of the cause of the wound. Levels of 200 mg/dl or more can impair the function of white blood cells (WBCs), which help prevent infection and are important in wound healing.

High blood glucose levels can prevent white blood cells like us from doing our job — preventing infection.

Hydration

Be sure to closely monitor and optimize the patient's hydration status — successful healing depends on it. Skin and subcutaneous tissues need to be well hydrated from the inside. Dehydration impairs the healing process by slowing the body's metabolism. Dehydration also reduces skin turgor, leaving skin vulnerable to new wounds.

Nutrition

Nutritional status helps you determine the patient's vulnerability to skin breakdown as well as the body's overall ability to heal. A comprehensive assessment of your patient's nutritional status also helps you plan effective care. (See *Parts of a nutritional assessment.*)

Keep in mind that nutrition is complex. If your assessment leads you to believe that the patient's nutritional status places him at risk for skin damage or for delayed wound healing, collaborate with a dietitian to develop the best possible treatment plan.

Blood albumin levels

Blood albumin levels are an essential factor in wound assessment for two important reasons:

First, skin is primarily constructed of protein, and albumin is a protein. If albumin levels are low, the body lacks an important building block for skin repair.

Second, albumin is the blood component that provides colloid osmotic pressure — the force that prevents fluid from leaking out of blood vessels into nearby tissues. (See *A closer look at albumin.*) If albumin levels fall below 3.5 g/dl, the patient can develop edema (fluid leakage into tissues), which compromises

Parts of a nutritional assessment

A comprehensive nutritional assessment can play an important part in wound care. Remember the four parts of a nutritional assessment, shown here.

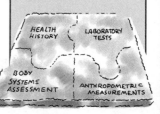

HEALTH HISTORY   LABORATORY TESTS

BODY SYSTEMS ASSESSMENT   ANTHROPOMETRIC MEASUREMENTS

wound healing. The patient also risks developing hypotension (low blood pressure) as fluid leaks out of the bloodstream into tissues. If blood pressure falls to the point where adequate blood flow is no longer maintained through the capillaries near the wound, healing slows or stops.

Oxygen and vascular supply

Healing requires oxygen—it's that simple. Therefore, anything that impedes full oxygenation also impedes healing. Your assessment should consider any factor with the potential to reduce the amount of oxygen available for healing. Possible problems include:
• impaired gas exchange, causing decreased oxygen levels in the blood
• hemoglobin levels too low to transport adequate oxygen
• low blood pressure that fails to drive oxygenated blood through capillaries
• insufficient arterial and capillary supply in the area of the wound.
　Any of these problems, or a combination of these problems, can deprive the wound of the oxygen needed for successful healing.

Smoke bomb

Smoking is a modifiable factor that impedes oxygenation of the wound. If your patient is a smoker, explain to him these ways in which smoking affects wound healing:
• Nicotine is a powerful vasoconstrictor that narrows peripheral blood vessels, thereby compromising blood flow to the skin.
• Because it's easier for hemoglobin to bind to the carbon monoxide present in cigarette smoke than it is for it to bind to oxygen, the blood that does squeeze through carries far less oxygen than it should.
• Lung tissue damaged by smoke doesn't function as well as it should, resulting in decreased oxygenation.

Pain

In order to promote patient comfort, you should control your patient's pain to the best of your ability. However, pain control has a practical purpose as well. In response to pain, the body releases epinephrine, a powerful vasoconstrictor. Vasoconstriction reduces blood flow to the wound. When you relieve pain, vasoconstriction subsides, blood vessels dilate, and blood flow to the wound improves.

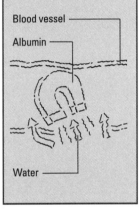

A closer look at albumin

Albumin, a large protein molecule, acts like a magnet to attract water and hold it inside the blood vessel.

Blood vessel
Albumin
Water

Make your patient aware of the ways in which smoking cessation facilitates wound healing but try to be tactful. It may help make him want to kick the habit.

Considering the cause

At some point in each assessment, focus on the cause of the wound to help ensure that you consider all factors that can influence healing. For instance, if you're assessing a patient with a venous insufficiency ulcer, you should measure the wound, of course. However, you should also measure calf circumference regularly to determine if efforts to reduce edema are succeeding. The best interventions for a venous insufficiency ulcer won't heal the wound if edema is left unchecked.

Diabetic details

Similarly, if you're assessing the wound of the patient with diabetes, check to make sure that his blood glucose is well controlled and that the calluses that tend to build up around diabetic foot ulcers are removed regularly. Otherwise, healing will be impeded.

In other words, don't miss the forest for the trees. As you focus on specific wound characteristics and how to describe them and track the healing process, never lose sight of the big picture.

Wound classification

The words you choose to describe your observations of a specific wound have to communicate the same thing to other members of the health care team, insurance companies, regulators, the patient's family, and ultimately the patient himself. This is a tall order when you consider that even wound care experts debate the descriptive phrases they use. Slough or eschar? Undermining or tunneling? How much drainage is "moderate"? Is the color green or yellow?

The best way to classify wounds is to use the basic system described here, which focuses on three categories of fundamental characteristics:
- wound age
- wound depth
- wound color.

It takes more than just time to determine whether a wound is acute or chronic.

Wound age

When determining the age of a wound, you need to first determine if the wound is acute or chronic. However, this determination can present a problem if you adhere solely to a time line. For instance, just how long is it before an acute wound becomes a chronic wound?

A different way of thinking

Rather than base your determination solely on time, consider a wound an acute wound if it's new or making progress as expected and a chronic wound any wound that isn't healing in a timely fashion. The main idea is that, in a chronic wound, healing has slowed or stopped and the wound is no longer getting smaller and shallower. Even if the wound bed appears healthy, red, and moist, if healing fails to progress, consider it a chronic wound.

More bad than good

Chronic wounds don't heal as easily as acute wounds. The drainage in chronic wounds contains a greater amount of destructive enzymes, and fibroblasts—the cells that function as the architects in wound healing—seem to lose their "oomph." They're less effective at producing collagen, divide less often, and send fewer signals to other cells telling them to divide and fill the wound. In other words, the wound changes from one that's vigorous and ready to heal, to one that's downright lazy!

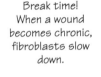

Break time! When a wound becomes chronic, fibroblasts slow down.

Wound depth

Wound depth is another fundamental characteristic used to classify wounds. In your assessment, record wound depth as partial-thickness or full-thickness. (See *Classifying wound depth*, page 32.)

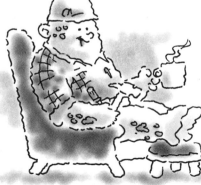

Partial-thickness

Partial-thickness wounds normally heal very quickly because they involve only the epidermal layer of the skin or extend through the epidermis into (but not through) the dermis. The dermis remains at least partially intact to generate the new epidermis needed to close the wound. Partial-thickness wounds are also less susceptible to infection because part of the body's first level of defense (the skin) is still intact. These wounds tend to be painful, however, and need protection from the air to reduce pain.

Full-thickness

Full-thickness wounds penetrate completely through the skin into underlying tissues. The wound may expose adipose tissue (fat), muscle, tendon, or bone. In the abdomen, you may see adipose tissue or omentum (the covering of the bowel). If the omentum is penetrated, the bowel may protrude through the wound (evisceration). Granulation tissue may be visible if the wound has started to heal.

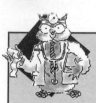

Get wise to wounds

Classifying wound depth

Wounds are classified as partial-thickness or full-thickness according to the depth of the wound. Partial-thickness wounds involve only the epidermis or extend into the dermis but not through it. Full-thickness wounds extend through the dermis into tissues beneath and may expose adipose tissue, muscle, or bone. The diagrams below illustrate the relative depth of both classifications.

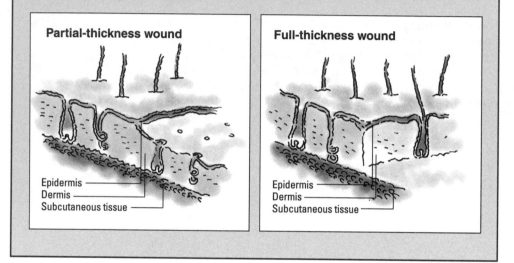

Partial-thickness wound

Epidermis
Dermis
Subcutaneous tissue

Full-thickness wound

Epidermis
Dermis
Subcutaneous tissue

Full-thickness wounds heal by granulation and contraction, which require more body resources and more time than the healing of partial-thickness wounds. When assessing a full-thickness wound, report the depth as well as the length and width of the wound.

The added pressure of pressure ulcers

In the case of pressure ulcers, wound depth allows you to stage the ulcer according to the classification system developed by the National Pressure Ulcer Advisory Panel (NPUAP). (See chapter 6, Pressure ulcers.)

Wound color

Wounds are also classified by the color of the wound bed. Wound color helps the wound care team determine whether debridement is appropriate. (See *Tailoring wound care to wound color.*)

Be picky about wound bed color! Only red will do, and the best shade is blood red — not pale pink or grayish red. There are liter-

Get wise to wounds

Tailoring wound care to wound color

With any wound, you can promote healing by keeping the wound moist, clean, and free from debris. For open wounds, using wound color can guide the specific management approach to aid healing.

Wound color	Management technique
Red	• Cover the wound, keep it moist and clean, and protect it from trauma. • Use a transparent dressing (such as Tegaderm or OpSite) over a gauze dressing moistened with normal saline solution, or use a hydrogel, foam, or hydrocolloid dressing to insulate and protect the wound.
Yellow	• Clean the wound and remove the yellow layer. • Cover the wound with a moisture-retentive dressing such as a hydrogel or foam dressing or a moist gauze dressing with or without a debriding enzyme. • Consider hydrotherapy with whirlpool or pulsatile lavage.
Black	• Debride the wound as ordered. Use an enzyme product (such as Accuzyme or Panafil), conservative sharp debridement, or hydrotherapy with whirlpool or pulsatile lavage. • For wounds with inadequate blood supply and noninfected heel ulcers, don't debride. Keep them clean and dry.

ally thousands of words to describe colors; however, you can simplify your assessment by sticking to the Red-Yellow-Black Classification System. This system is a useful tool for developing effective wound care management plans.

Red means you're ahead

If the wound bed is red (the color of healthy granulation tissue) the wound is healthy and normal healing is under way. When a wound begins to heal, a layer of pale pink granulation tissue covers the wound bed. As this layer thickens, it becomes beefy red.

Mellow yellow

If the wound bed is yellow, beware! A yellow color in the wound bed may be a film of fibrin on the tissue. Fibrin is a sticky substance that normally acts as a glue in tissue rebuilding. However, if the wound is unhealthy or too dry, fibrin builds up into a layer that can't be rinsed off and may require debridement. Tissue that has recently died due to ischemia or infection also may be yellow and must be debrided.

Black = debridement

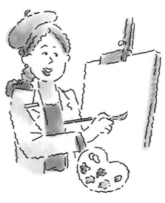

Remember to classify wounds according to the least healthy color present.

If the wound bed is black, be alarmed. A black wound bed signals necrosis (tissue death). Eschar (dead, avascular tissue) covers the wound, slowing the healing process and providing microorganisms with a site in which to proliferate. When eschar covers a wound, accurate assessment of wound depth is difficult and should be deferred until eschar is removed.

Typically, debridement is indicated for black wounds; however, ulcers caused by ischemia (damage due to inadequate blood supply) and uninfected heel pressure ulcers are exceptions. Ischemic wounds won't heal until blood supply is improved, and they're less likely to become infected if kept dry. The wound can be debrided and kept moist after blood supply is reestablished. (The body can then fend off infection and heal the wound.) As long as they're uninfected, heel pressure ulcers tend to heal from beneath the ulcer and don't require debridement.

Multicolored wounds

If you note two or even all three colors in a wound, classify the wound according to the least healthy color present. For example, if your patient's wound appears both red and yellow, classify it as a yellow wound.

Wound assessment

Gathering information about a wound requires you to use almost all of your senses. Be sure to assess drainage, the wound bed, and patient pain. Assess the wound bed and the surrounding skin only after they have been cleaned. Remember as you perform your assessment that it doesn't matter what method you use to record your observations, it's just important to be consistent.

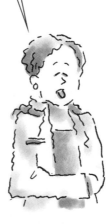

Assessing a wound requires you to use all of your senses — well, almost all of them. I wouldn't recommend tasting.

Assessing drainage

To begin collecting information about wound drainage, inspect the dressing as it's removed and record answers to such questions as:
• Is the drainage well contained, or is it oozing from the edges? If it's oozing, consider using a more absorbent dressing.
• In the case of an occlusive dressing, were the dressing edges well sealed? (A hydrocolloid in the gluteal cleft area becomes a

greenhouse for bacteria if the edges are loose.) If the patient has fecal incontinence, it's even more important to note the seal status.
• Is the dressing saturated or dry?
• How much drainage is there: a scant, moderate, or large amount?
• What are the color and consistency of the drainage? (See *Drainage descriptors.*)

Skipping the swab?

Also consider the texture of the drainage. If the drainage has a thick, creamy texture, the wound contains an excessive amount of bacteria. However, this doesn't necessarily mean a clinically significant infection is present. Document the characteristics of the drainage. Drainage might be creamy because it contains WBCs that have killed bacteria. The drainage is also contaminated with surface bacteria that naturally live in moist environments on the human body. Because of this bacterial colonization, guidelines developed by the Agency for Health Care Policy and Research, now the Agency for Healthcare Research and Quality, recommend against using swab cultures to identify wound infections. Nonetheless, some doctors

---

Get wise to wounds

Drainage descriptors

The chart below provides terminology that you can use to describe the color and consistency of wound drainage.

Description	Color and consistency
Serous	• Clear or light yellow • Thin and watery
Sanguinous	• Red (with fresh blood) • Thin
Serosan-guinous	• Pink to light red • Thin • Watery
Purulent	• Creamy yellow, green, white, or tan • Thick and opaque

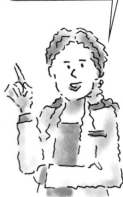

Keep in mind that you should check the dressing as it's removed, but check the wound and skin only after they have been cleaned.

still order swab cultures because they're easy to collect and inexpensive.

Ideally, obtain a swab of the clear fluid expressed from the wound tissue after it has been thoroughly cleaned. This is more likely to produce a sample of the bacteria in question. Punch biopsy of tissue or needle aspiration of fluid may also be used. These methods require more skill but are more likely to reveal accurate results.

Assessing the wound bed

As you assess the wound bed, record information about:
- wound dimensions, including size and depth
- tunneling and undermining
- bed texture and moisture
- wound odor
- margins and surrounding skin.

Dimensions

Because accurately recording wound dimensions is important, many health care facilities use photography as a tool in wound assessment. If photography is available in your facility, it should be included in your assessment of wound characteristics. Some photographic techniques produce a picture with a grid overlay that's useful for measuring. Remember, however, that there are qualities of the wound that a camera simply can't record. (See *What's missing?*)

Get out your ruler

The most common method of measuring wound dimensions is to use a tape measure. Make sure it's a disposable device to prevent contamination and cross-contamination. Record the length of the wound as the longest overall distance across the wound (regardless of orientation), and record the width as the longest measurement perpendicular (at a right angle) to your length measurement. (See *Measuring a wound*, page 38.)

Be sure to record any observed areas of discoloration of the intact skin around the wound opening separately—not as part of the wound bed. Record all measurements in centimeters.

Trace the wound

Another way to measure the wound is to use wound tracing (wound margins are traced on a sheet of clear plastic). You use the tracing to calculate an approximate wound area. This method provides only a rough estimate but is simple and fairly quick.

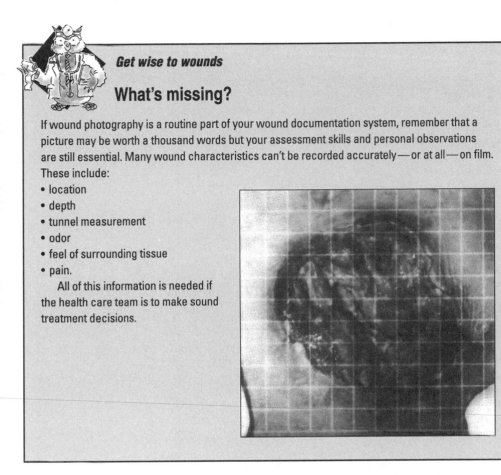

Get wise to wounds

What's missing?

If wound photography is a routine part of your wound documentation system, remember that a picture may be worth a thousand words but your assessment skills and personal observations are still essential. Many wound characteristics can't be recorded accurately—or at all—on film. These include:

- location
- depth
- tunnel measurement
- odor
- feel of surrounding tissue
- pain.

    All of this information is needed if the health care team is to make sound treatment decisions.

How deep

To measure the depth of the wound, you'll need a cotton-tipped swab. Gently insert the swab into the deepest portion of the wound and then carefully mark the stick where it meets the edge of the skin. Remove the swab and measure the distance from your mark to the end to determine depth.

Tunneling and undermining

It's also important to measure tunnels, or sinus tracts (extensions of the wound bed into adjacent tissue), and undermining (areas of the wound bed that extend under the skin). Measure these features just as you would the depth. Carefully insert a cotton-tipped swab to the bottom of the tunnel or to the end of the undermined area; then mark the stick and measure the distance from your mark to the end of the swab. If a tunnel is large, palpate it with a gloved finger rather than a swab because you can sense the end of the tunnel better with your finger. This also avoids damaging the tissue.

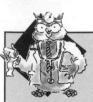

Measuring a wound

When measuring a wound, first determine the longest distance across the open area of the wound—regardless of orientation. In the photograph below, note the line used to illustrate this length.

A wound's width is simply the longest distance across the wound at a right angle to the length. Note the relationship of length and width in the photograph below. Also note the area of reddened, intact skin and white macerated skin. These areas would be measured and recorded as surrounding erythema and maceration—not as part of the wound itself. In this full-thickness ischial pressure ulcer, you would also record a depth and note any areas of tunneling or undermining.

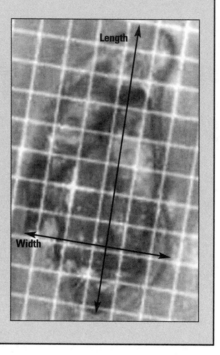

Texture

The texture of the wound bed provides just as much information about the wound and healing as its color. If you note very smooth red tissue in a partial-thickness wound, it's most likely the dermis. In a full-thickness wound, it's probably muscle tissue—not granulation tissue. In a full-thickness wound, healthy granulation tissue—which has a soft, bumpy appearance that's like the surface of a bowl of tapioca, only red—is a sign of proper healing.

Moisture

The wound bed should be moist—but not overly moist. Moisture allows the cells and chemicals needed for healing to move about the wound surface.

Desert storm

In dry wound beds, cells involved in healing, which normally exist in a fluid environment, are a bit like fish in a desert — they can't move. WBCs can't fight infection, enzymes like collagenase can't break down dead material, and macrophages can't carry away debris. The wound edges curl up to preserve moisture remaining in the edge and epithelial cells (new skin cells) fail to grow over and cover the wound. Healing grinds to a halt and necrotic tissue builds up.

Gasp! Dryness is a drag. If the wound bed is too dry, I can't move. This makes it hard for me to advance healing...

Flood watch

Too much moisture poses a different problem. It floods the wound and spills out onto the skin, where the constant moisture causes the death of skin cells.

Odor

If kept clean, a noninfected wound usually produces little, if any, odor. (One exception is the odor normally present under a hydrocolloid dressing that develops as a by-product of the degradation process.) A newly detected odor might be a sign of infection; record it in your findings and report it to the doctor. When documenting wound odor, it's important to include when the odor was noted and whether it went away with wound cleaning.

If an odor develops, it can present an embarrassing or otherwise uncomfortable situation for the patient as well as his family, guests, and roommate. If you notice an odor, or if your patient says he notices one, use an odor eliminator. Odor eliminators differ from air fresheners in that they aren't scents that mask odors but rather compounds that bind with, and neutralize, the molecules responsible for the odor.

...Make sure I'm not swimming either, though. Too much moisture can be the death of me.

Margins and surrounding skin

When assessing wound margins, you'll want to see skin that's smooth — not rolled — and tightly adherent to the wound bed. Rolled skin may indicate that the wound bed is too dry. Loose skin at the edges may indicate additional shearing injury (separation of skin layers), possibly due to a rough transfer or repositioning. In this case, improve transfer and repositioning techniques to prevent recurrence.

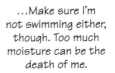

Rainbow connections

Sailors used to use the color of the sky to predict danger at sea. In a similar fashion, the color of the skin around the wound can alert you to impending problems that can impede healing:

• White skin indicates maceration, or too much moisture, and signals the need for a protective barrier around the wound and a more absorbent dressing.

• Red skin can indicate inflammation, injury (for example, tape burn, excessive pressure, or chemical exposure), or infection. Remember that inflammation is healthy only during the inflammatory phase of healing—not after!

• Purple skin can indicate bruising, one sign of trauma.

Let your fingers do the talking

Your fingers are invaluable tools you may be taking for granted. During your assessment of the area around the wound, your fingers will tell you much. For example, gently probe the tissue around the wound bed to determine if it's soft or hard (indurated). Indurated tissue, even in the absence of erythema (redness), is one indication of infection. Similarly, if your patient has dark skin, it may be impossible to see color cues. Again, your fingers can help. Probe the area around the wound bed and compare the feel to surrounding healthy skin. A tender area of skin that appears shiny and feels hard may indicate inflammation in such a patient.

Assessing pain

Assessing patient pain is an important part of wound assessment. You'll want to note not only pain associated with the injury itself but also pain associated with healing and with therapies employed to promote healing. To fully understand your patient's pain, talk with him and ask about his pain. Then, independently, watch to see how he responds to pain and the therapies provided. As always, remember to record your findings. (See *How to assess pain.*)

Listen and learn

If your patient is conscious and can communicate, have him rate his pain before and during each dressing change. If your notes reveal that his pain is higher before the dressing change, it may indicate an impending infection, even before any other signs appear.

If your patient says the dressing change itself is painful, you might consider administering pain medication before the procedure or changing the dressing technique itself. For example, if treatment calls for a wet-to-dry debridement technique, you can anticipate

How to assess pain

To properly assess patient pain, consider the patient's descriptions and your own observations of his reaction to pain and treatments.

Talk to your patient

Begin your pain assessment by asking your patient the following questions:

• Where is the pain located? How long does it last? How often does it occur?

• What does the pain feel like? (Let the patient describe it; don't prompt.)

• What relieves the pain? What makes it worse?

• How do you usually get relief?

• How would you rate your pain on a scale of 0 to 10, with 0 representing no pain and 10 representing the worst pain?

Talking with the patient about his pain in this manner helps him define his pain, for himself as well as you, and helps you evaluate the effectiveness of therapies used to relieve pain.

Monitor and observe your patient

As you work with the patient, observe his responses to pain and to interventions intended to relieve pain.

Behavioral responses to watch for include:

• altered body position

• moaning

• sighing

• grimacing

• withdrawing from painful stimuli

• crying

• restlessness

• muscle twitching

• immobility.

Sympathetic responses, normally associated with mild to moderate pain, include:

• pallor

• elevated blood pressure

• dilated pupils

• tension in skeletal muscles

• dyspnea (shortness of breath)

• tachycardia (rapid heart beat)

• diaphoresis (sweating).

Parasympathetic responses, which are more common in cases of severe, deep pain, include:

• pallor

• lower than normal blood pressure

• bradycardia (slower than normal heartbeat)

• nausea and vomiting

• weakness

• dizziness

• loss of consciousness.

that the patient will experience pain, and it makes sense to provide some measure of preprocedure pain medication. However, remember to document this pain and report it to the doctor. Less painful methods of removing dead tissue exist but, if the patient's pain isn't documented and communicated, wet-to-dry debridement orders may stand and the patient may suffer unnecessary discomfort.

Useful tips for removal

In general, when removing adherent dressings, it's less painful if you soak the dressing or, over intact skin, use an adhesive remover. Also, keep the skin taut. Press down on the skin to release the dressing, rather than just pulling the dressing off. If the patient still says that dressing removal is painful, the team may wish to choose a less adherent dressing type.

Wound documentation

In the course of a wound assessment, you amass quite a bit of useful information about the patient, his environment, the characteristics of his wound, and his current status in the healing process. In fact, your assessment has created a picture of the wound that accurately depicts your patient and his current status.

Picture this...

Use the mnemonic device WOUND PICTURE to help you recall and organize all of the key facts that should be included in your documentation:

Wound or ulcer location

Odor? (in room or just when wound is uncovered?)

Ulcer category, stage (for pressure ulcer) or classification (for diabetic ulcer), and depth (partial-thickness or full-thickness)

Necrotic tissue?

Dimension of wound (shape, length, width, depth); **D**rainage color, consistency, and amount (scant, moderate, large)

Pain? (when it occurs, what relieves it, patient's description, patient's rating on scale of 0 to 10)

Induration? (surrounding tissue hard or soft?)

Color of wound bed (red-yellow-black or combination)

Tunneling? (record length and direction—toward patient's right, left, head, feet)

Undermining? (record length and direction, using clock references to describe)

Redness or other discoloration in surrounding skin?

Edge of skin loose or tightly adhered? Edges flat or rolled under?

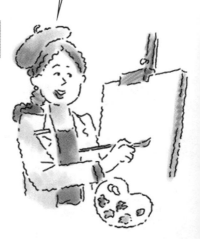

The picture of the wound that you paint during your initial assessment plays an important role in wound monitoring. It serves as a benchmark for wound healing.

Wound monitoring

The next step is to monitor the patient throughout the healing process, periodically reassessing his status and documenting progress to full healing. Not only is this an excellent way to determine progress and the usefulness of interventions but it's also now a requirement for some regulatory agencies such as the Centers for Medicare and Medicaid Services (CMS).

Your initial assessment sets the benchmark for subsequent monitoring and reassessment activities. One assessment is a static report. A series of assessments, however, becomes a moving picture illustrating the dynamic aspect of the healing process. In this way, all members of the health care team can see progress toward healing (or failure to thrive), developing complications, and the relative success of interventions. The view will depend on the accuracy, quality, and consistency of your documentation.

The prospect of monitoring, reassessing, and documenting over time may seem exciting or daunting, depending on your current energy level. But take heart. Several good research-based documentation tools are available — or your facility may have its own — to help you manage the task. Let's take a look.

Documentation tools

Most wound documentation tools in use in the United States focus on pressure ulcers. Pressure ulcers were selected as the basis because of the tremendous impact they have had on countless patients' lives and the health care system itself. Pressure ulcers are painful, typically chronic, life-disrupting, and expensive to treat — both in dollars and in amount of time spent by providers. They're also preventable.

Pressure Ulcer Scale for Healing

The Pressure Ulcer Scale for Healing (PUSH) tool was developed and revised by NPUAP and is only applicable to pressure ulcers. (See *PUSH tool*, page 44.)

When working with this tool, you develop three scores: one for the surface area (length × width), one for the drainage amount, and one for the tissue type in the wound during each review. The sum of these scores yields a total score for the wound on a given day. This score is then plotted on a pressure ulcer healing record and healing graph. By recording and reviewing scores over time, you can determine the pace of progress toward healing.

NPUAP is working with CMS to incorporate the PUSH tool into the Minimum Data Set, a required documentation form in long-term care facilities.

Pressure Sore Status Tool

The Pressure Sore Status Tool (PSST) allows you to track scores for eleven factors over time. These factors are each scored based on a number scale, and the scores are added. The total score reflects overall wound status.

PUSH tool

The beauty of the Pressure Ulcer Scale for Healing (PUSH) tool is its simplicity. It's quick and easy to score.

Patient name _David Quinn_   User location _Sunview Nursing Home_

Patient I.D. # _0162386_   Date _1/3/03_

Directions

Observe and measure the pressure ulcer. Categorize the ulcer with respect to surface area, exudate, and type of wound tissue. Record a subscore for each of the ulcer characteristics. Add the subscores to obtain the total score. A comparison of total scores measured over time provides an indication of the improvement or deterioration in pressure ulcer healing.

Length	0	1	2	3	4	5	
× width	0 cm²	< 0.3 cm²	0.3 to 0.6 cm²	0.7 to 1.0 cm²	1.1 to 2.0 cm²	2.1 to 3.0 cm²	Subscore
	6	**7**	**8**	**9**	**10**		
	3.1 to 4.0 cm²	4.1 to 8.0 cm²	8.1 to 12.0 cm²	12.1 to 24.0 cm²	> 24.0 cm²		3
Exudate amount	**0** None	**1** Light	**2** Moderate	**3** Heavy			Subscore 1
Tissue type	**0** Closed	**1** Epithelial tissue	**2** Granulation tissue	**3** Slough	**4** Necrotic tissue		Subscore 1
						Total score:	5

Length × width

Measure the greatest length (head-to-toe) and the greatest width (side-to-side) using a centimeter ruler. Multiply these two measurements (length × width) to obtain an estimate of surface area in square centimeters (cm²). Don't guess! Always use a centimeter ruler and always use the same method each time the ulcer is measured.

Exudate amount

Estimate the amount of exudate (drainage) present after removal of the dressing and before applying any topical agent to the ulcer. Estimate the exudate as none, light, moderate, or heavy.

Tissue type

This refers to the types of tissue that are present in the wound (ulcer) bed. Score as a 4 if necrotic tissue is present. Score as a 3 if slough is present and necrotic tissue is absent. Score as a 2 if the wound is clean and contains granulation tissue. Score a superficial wound that's reepithelializing as a 1. When the wound is closed, score it as a 0.

4—Necrotic tissue (eschar): Black, brown, or tan tissue that adheres firmly to the wound bed or ulcer edges and may be either firmer or softer than surrounding tissue

3—Slough: Yellow or white tissue that adheres to the ulcer bed in strings or thick clumps or is mucinous

2—Granulation tissue: Pink or beefy red tissue with a shiny, moist, granular appearance

1—Epithelial tissue: For superficial ulcers, new pink or shiny tissue (skin) that grows in from the edges or as islands on the ulcer surface

0—Closed or resurfaced: Completely covered wound with epithelium (new skin)

Adapted with permission from PUSH tool version 3.0, © 1998 National Pressure Ulcer Advisory Panel, Reston, Va.

The PSST is a precise record of wound changes and is fairly time consuming to fill out. Consequently, it's used more in research than in clinical practice.

Wound Healing Scale

The Wound Healing Scale is a simple classification system that combines a designation for wound stage, or thickness, with a tissue descriptor. For example, a stage 3 pressure ulcer containing necrotic tissue is recorded as 3N. Using this tool, you can track the general direction of healing by noting, for example, that this week the wound is an FG (full-thickness with granulation tissue), whereas last week it was an FN (full-thickness with necrotic tissue). The tool includes modifiers that permit you to use it for all types of wounds, although it was developed initially for use with pressure ulcers.

Sussman Wound Healing Tool

The Sussman Wound Healing Tool was developed to help physical therapists track pressure ulcer healing. This tool lists 10 wound attributes and classifies each as "good" or "not good" in terms of wound healing. For example, granulation tissue is classified "good" and undermining is classified "not good." During each assessment, record your findings for each of the 10 attributes that apply to your patient; over time, this provides a picture of healing or failure to thrive.

Recognizing complications

It's important to monitor and track, or reassess, wound status to identify signs and symptoms of complications or failure to thrive as early in the process as possible. Early intervention improves the likelihood of resolving complications successfully and getting the healing process back on track.

Oh say, can you see?

You'll conduct your reassessments using the same criteria used in the initial assessment, with one added advantage—perspective. Careful monitoring can help you catch failure to thrive early so you can intervene appropriately. (See *Recognizing failure to thrive*, pages 46 and 47.)

The sooner, the better

Success or failure of the healing process has a tremendous impact on the patient's quality of life as well as his

> In wound care, you may be able to foresee problems by recognizing signs of complications or failure to thrive.

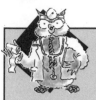

Get wise to wounds

Recognizing failure to thrive

This chart presents the most common signs of failure to thrive as well as associated probable causes and appropriate interventions.

Sign	Cause	Intervention
Wound bed		
Too dry	• Exposure of tissue and cells normally in a moist environment to air • Inadequate hydration	• Add moisture regularly. • Use a dressing that maintains moisture such as a hydrocolloid or hydrogel dressing.
No change in size or depth for 2 weeks	• Pressure or trauma to the area • Poor nutrition, poor circulation, inadequate hydration, or medications • Poor control of disease processes such as diabetes • Inadequate pain control • Infection	• Reassess the patient for local or systemic problems that impair wound healing, and intervene as necessary.
Increase in size or depth	• Debridement • Ischemia due to excess pressure or poor circulation • Infection	• If debridement of necrotic tissue is being done, no intervention is necessary. (This is normal.) • Poor circulation may not be resolvable, but consider adding warmth to the area and administering a vasodilator or antiplatelet medication.
Necrosis	• Ischemia	• Perform debridement if the remaining living tissue has adequate circulation.
Increase in drainage or change of drainage color from clear to purulent	• Infection • Autolytic or enzymatic debridement	• No intervention is necessary if caused by autolytic or enzymatic debridement. Increase in drainage or change of drainage color is expected because of the breakdown of dead tissue. • If debridement isn't the cause, assess the wound for infection.
Tunneling	• Pressure over bony prominences • Presence of foreign body • Deep infection	• Protect the area from pressure. • Irrigate and inspect the tunnel as carefully as possible for a hidden suture or leftover bit of dressing material. • If the tunnel doesn't shorten in length each week, thoroughly clean and obtain a tissue biopsy for infection and, with a chronic wound, for possible malignancy.

Recognizing failure to thrive (continued)

Sign	Cause	Intervention
Wound edges		
Red, hot skin; tenderness; and induration	• Inflammation due to excess pressure or infection	• If pressure relief doesn't resolve the inflammation within 24 hours, topical antimicrobial therapy may be indicated.
White skin (maceration)	• Excess moisture	• Protect the skin with petrolatum ointment or barrier wipe. • If practical, obtain an order for a more absorptive dressing.
Rolled skin edges	• Too-dry wound bed	• Obtain an order for moisture-retentive dressings. • If rolling isn't resolved in 1 week, debridement of the edges may be necessary.
Undermining or ecchymosis of surrounding skin (loose or bruised skin edges)	• Excess shearing force to the area	• Initiate measures to protect the area, especially during patient transfers.

family's quality of life. Early intervention can mean that a patient with a diabetic foot ulcer can avoid amputation or a paraplegic patient with an ischial ulcer can once again sit up and lead an active life.

Chronic ulcers pose a particularly difficult problem, not only for individual practitioners but also for the health care industry as a whole. Treating chronic ulcers is expensive because they're difficult or impossible to heal. Consequently, the people footing the largest portion of the bill—the government and insurance companies—are placing increased emphasis on early intervention and prevention.

Winning in wound healing

Now that you know what to look for when things *aren't* going well, let's take a look at what you can expect to see when healing is progressing smoothly. In this case, your patient:
• is well hydrated, well nourished, comfortable, and warm
• is well managed for associated or contributing diseases, such as diabetes, heart failure, or renal failure
• exhibits normal immune system response.

In addition, the wound itself:
• receives the oxygen and nutrients it needs (adequate vascular supply)
• is moist and protected from the environment
• is free from necrotic tissue.

These conditions optimize wound healing. By using the assessment techniques presented in this chapter, you'll be a part of this success.

Star player

Wound healing isn't a simple matter to coordinate. Through vigilance and consistent assessment and documentation, success is much more likely. By using most of your senses, you can have a tremendous influence on whether a wound heals or becomes chronic and harder to manage. Recognizing red flags that warn of failure to thrive, and knowing the appropriate interventions, make you a part of the winning wound healing team!

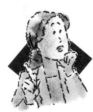

Quick quiz

1. A wound that extends through the epidermis and part way into the dermis is classified as a:

    A.   chronic wound.
    B.   acute wound.
    C.   partial-thickness wound.
    D.   full-thickness wound.

Answer: C. Partial-thickness wounds extend into but not through the dermis, which retains function that helps the healing process.

2. Which wound bed color indicates normal, healthy granulation tissue?

    A.   Red
    B.   Yellow
    C.   Tan
    D.   Black

Answer: A. Red tissue in a wound bed indicates healthy granulation tissue.

3. If you see multiple colors in a wound bed, you should classify the wound according to the:

A. healthiest color you see.
B. least healthy color you see.
C. color most visible.
D. color least visible.

Answer: B. Using the Red-Yellow-Black Classification System, you should classify a wound with multiple colors according to the least healthy color you see.

4. Wound healing is facilitated by:
A. a dark environment.
B. exposure to air.
C. a dry environment.
D. a moist environment.

Answer: D. Moisture in the wound bed allows the cells and chemicals needed for healing to move across the wound surface.

5. The PUSH tool is useful for:
A. measuring the size of a pressure ulcer.
B. detecting wound infection.
C. tracking pressure ulcer healing.
D. measuring the depth of a pressure ulcer.

Answer: C. The PUSH tool allows you to track pressure ulcer healing.

6. Which term could be used to accurately describe drainage that's thin and bright red?
A. Serous
B. Sanguinous
C. Serosanguinous
D. Purulent

Answer: B. Sanguinous drainage is red, usually due to the presence of fresh blood.

7. Which is an appropriate intervention for a wound that has tunneling?
A. Provide warmth to the area.
B. Perform conservative sharp debridement.
C. Protect the area from pressure.
D. No intervention is necessary.

Answer: C. Because tunneling may be caused by pressure over bony prominences, the wound should be protected from pressure.

Scoring

☆☆☆ If you answered all seven questions correctly, stand up and bow. You're a wound care all-star!

☆☆ If you answered four to six questions correctly, great job. You're a cut above the rest.

☆ If you answered fewer than four questions correctly, don't worry. You've just skinned the surface of wound care; there are eight more chapters to go!

Basic wound care procedures

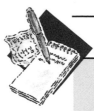

Just the facts

In this chapter, you'll learn:

♦ the components of a wound care order

♦ basic wound care procedures

♦ six basic types of dressings.

A look at wound care orders

Wound care orders are typically written by doctors, podiatrists, nurse practitioners, and physician assistants. However, policies and procedures related to skin and wound care activities are commonly written by and carried out by registered nurses. The doctor in charge reviews and approves these policies and procedures. Many facilities now have specific policies and procedures for different types of wounds.

What should be included in wound care orders

When you're presented with an order to provide wound care, or if you're in the position to write wound policies and procedures, keep in mind the following list of essential information that you should include:

• wound description, including cause, location, appearance, and size
• cleaning agent and method to be used
• type of dressing for the primary and, if needed, secondary layers
• topical medications needed
• frequency of dressing changes
• time frame for evaluating and changing dressings.

Typically, if there's no change in the wound in 2 weeks, the patient's condition and wound should be reassessed and the management plan should be revised accordingly. New orders may be

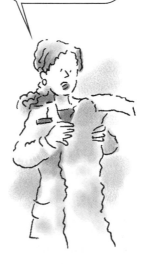

Making a list and checking it twice...Make sure that wound care orders contain all of the necessary information.

Get wise to wounds

Guide to making wound care decisions

Ask yourself the following questions to help you determine what kind of care your patient's wound needs and how you should proceed.

How should I clean the wound?
___Water ___Saline ___ Commercial wound cleaner

Assess the wound and document according to facility policy and procedure.

Is the wound clean or necrotic?
___Clean ___Necrotic

Is gangrene present?
___Wet ___Dry

Is there blood flow to the area?
___Yes ___No

Does the wound need debridement?
___Yes ___No

Is the wound infected?
___Yes ___No

What kind of debridement is appropriate?
___Sharp ___Chemical ___Mechanical ___Autolytic

Is the wound partial-thickness or full-thickness?
___Partial ___Full

How much drainage is present?
___None ___Minimal ___Moderate ___Heavy

How does the surrounding skin appear?
___Intact ___Irritated ___Denuded

What cover or dressing is appropriate?
___Transparent film ___Hydrogel ___Hydrocolloid ___Alginate ___Foam
___Gauze ___Other

needed. If no healing progress is apparent after 4 to 12 weeks of treatment, referral to a wound care specialist is recommended.

Determining a wound care plan

Wound care is an art and a science. It's based on the whole patient: his condition, his needs, and the wound profile. The goals of wound care include:

* promoting wound healing by controlling or eliminating causative factors
* preventing or managing infection
* removing nonviable tissue (debridement) as needed
* enhancing adequate blood supply
* providing nutritional and fluid support
* establishing and maintaining a clean, moist, protected wound bed
* managing wound fluid or drainage
* maintaining the skin surrounding the wound to ensure it remains dry and intact.

With any wound, healing may be promoted by keeping the wound moist, clean, and free from debris. However, requirements for providing wound care vary according to the patient assessment and the nature of the wound. (See *Guide to making wound care decisions.*)

Basic wound care

Basic wound care centers on cleaning and dressing the wound. Because open wounds are colonized (or contaminated) with bacteria, observe clean technique using clean, nonsterile gloves during wound care unless sterile dressing changes are specified. Always follow standard precautions.

The goal of wound cleaning is to remove debris and contaminants from the wound without damaging healthy tissue. The wound should be cleaned initially; repeat cleaning as needed or before a new dressing is applied.

The basic purpose of a dressing, to provide an optimal environment in which the body can heal itself, should be considered before one is selected. Functions of a wound dressing include:

* protecting the wound from contamination and trauma
* providing compression if bleeding or swelling is anticipated
* applying medications
* absorbing drainage or debrided necrotic tissue
* filling or packing the wound
* protecting the skin surrounding the wound.

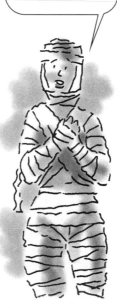

No need to keep it under wraps. Everyone should know that basic wound care involves cleaning and dressing the wound.

The cardinal rule is to keep moist tissue moist and dry tissue dry. Ideally, a dressing should keep the wound moist, absorb drainage or debris, conform to the wound, and be adhesive to surrounding skin yet also be easily removable. It should also be user-friendly, require minimal changes, decrease the need for a secondary dressing layer, and be cost-effective and comfortable for the patient.

What you need

Hypoallergenic tape or elastic netting ❀ overbed table ❀ piston-type irrigating system ❀ two pairs of gloves ❀ cleaning solution (such as normal saline solution) as ordered ❀ sterile 4″ × 4″ gauze pads ❀ selected topical dressing ❀ linen-saver pads ❀ impervious plastic trash bag ❀ disposable wound-measuring device

Getting ready

Assemble the equipment at the patient's bedside. Use clean or sterile technique, depending on facility policy and wound care orders. Cut tape into strips for securing dressings. Loosen lids on cleaning solutions and medications for easy removal. Attach an impervious plastic trash bag to the overbed table to hold used dressings and refuse.

How you do it

• Before any dressing change, wash your hands and review the principles of standard precautions.

Cleaning the wound

• Provide privacy, and explain the procedure to the patient to allay his fears and promote cooperation.
• Position the patient in a way that maximizes his comfort while allowing easy access to the wound site.
• Cover bed linens with a linen-saver pad to prevent soiling.

No splashing

• Open the cleaning solution container and carefully pour cleaning solution into a bowl to avoid splashing. The bowl may be clean or sterile, depending on facility policy. (See *Choosing a cleaning agent.*)
• Open the packages of supplies.
• Put on gloves.

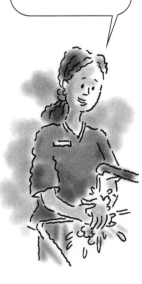

Before any dressing change, be sure to wash your hands. Follow standard precautions during the procedure.

Get wise to wounds

Choosing a cleaning agent

The most commonly used cleaning agent is sterile normal saline solution, which provides a moist environment, promotes granulation tissue formation, and causes minimal fluid shifts in healthy adults.

Antiseptic solutions may damage tissue and delay healing but are sometimes used for cleaning infected or newly contaminated wounds. Examples of antiseptic solutions include:

• *hydrogen peroxide* (commonly used half-strength), which irrigates the wound and aids in mechanical debridement (its foaming action also warms the wound, promoting vasodilation and reducing inflammation)

• *acetic acid,* which treats *Pseudomonas* infection

• *sodium hypochlorite* (Dakin's fluid), an antiseptic that also slightly dissolves necrotic tissue (this unstable solution must be freshly prepared every 24 hours)

• *povidone-iodine,* a broad-spectrum, fast-acting antimicrobial agent (watch for patient sensitivity to this solution; also, protect the surrounding skin from contact because this solution can dry and stain the skin).

• Gently roll or lift an edge of the soiled dressing to obtain a starting point. Support adjacent skin while gently releasing the soiled dressing from the skin. When possible, remove the dressing in the direction of hair growth.

• Discard the soiled dressing and your contaminated gloves in the impervious plastic trash bag to avoid contaminating the clean or sterile field.

• Put on a clean pair of gloves (sterile or nonsterile, depending on facility policy or the wound care order).

• Inspect the wound. Note the color, amount, and odor of drainage and necrotic debris.

• Fold a sterile 4″ × 4″ gauze pad into quarters and grasp it with your fingers. Make sure the folded edge faces outward.

• Dip the folded gauze into the cleaning solution. Alternatively, use a wound cleaning solution in a spray gun bottle.

Circles on the skin

• When cleaning, be sure to move from the least-contaminated area to the most-contaminated area. For a linear shaped wound, such as an incision, gently wipe from top to bottom in one motion, starting directly over the wound and moving outward. For an open wound, such as a pressure ulcer, gently wipe in concentric circles, again starting directly over the wound and moving outward.

• Discard the gauze pad in the plastic trash bag.

• Using a clean gauze pad for each wiping motion, repeat the procedure until you've cleaned the entire wound.
• Dry the wound with 4″ × 4″ gauze pads, using the same procedure as for cleaning. Discard the used gauze pads in the plastic trash bag.
• Measure the perimeter of the wound with a disposable wound-measuring device (for example, a square, transparent card with concentric circles arranged in bull's-eye fashion and bordered with a straight-edge ruler). Measure the longest length and the widest width.
• Measure the depth of a full-thickness wound. Insert a sterile cotton-tipped applicator gently into the deepest part of the wound bed and place a mark on the applicator where it meets the skin level. Measure the marked applicator to determine wound depth.

Testing for tunneling

• Gently probe the wound bed and edges with your finger or a sterile cotton-tipped applicator to assess for wound tunneling or undermining. Tunneling usually signals wound extension along fascial planes. Gauge tunnel depth by determining how far you can insert your finger or the cotton-tipped applicator.
• Next, reassess the condition of the skin and wound. Note the character of the clean wound bed and the surrounding skin.
• If you observe adherent necrotic material, notify a wound care specialist or a doctor to ensure appropriate debridement.
• Prepare to apply the appropriate topical dressing. Instructions for applying topical moist saline gauze, hydrocolloid, transparent, alginate, foam, and hydrogel dressings follow. (See *Choosing a wound dressing.*) For other dressings or topical agents, follow your facility's protocol or the manufacturer's instructions.

Applying a moist saline gauze dressing

• Moisten the gauze dressing with normal saline solution. Wring out excess fluid.
• Gently place the dressing into the wound surface. To separate surfaces within the wound, gently guide the gauze between opposing wound surfaces. To avoid damage to tissues, don't pack the gauze tightly.
• To protect the surrounding skin from moisture, apply a sealant or barrier.
• Change the dressing often enough to keep the wound moist.

Applying a hydrocolloid dressing

• Choose a clean, dry, presized dressing, or cut one to overlap the wound by about 1″ (2.5 cm). Remove the dressing from its pack-

Dress for success

Choosing a wound dressing

The patient's needs and wound characteristics determine which type of dressing to use on a wound.

Gauze dressings
Made of absorptive cotton or synthetic fabric, gauze dressings are permeable to water, water vapor, and oxygen and may be impregnated with hydrogel or another agent. When uncertain about which dressing to use, you may apply a gauze dressing moistened in saline solution until a wound specialist recommends definitive treatment.

Hydrocolloid dressings
Hydrocolloid dressings are adhesive, moldable wafers made of a carbohydrate-based material and usually have waterproof backings. They're impermeable to oxygen, water, and water vapor, and most have some absorptive properties.

Transparent film dressings
Transparent film dressings are clear, adherent, and nonabsorptive. These polymer-based dressings are permeable to oxygen and water vapor but not to water. Their transparency allows visual inspection. Because they can't absorb drainage, they're used on partial-thickness wounds with minimal exudate.

Alginate dressings
Made from seaweed, alginate dressings are nonwoven, absorptive dressings available as soft white sterile pads or ropes. They absorb excessive exudate and may be used on infected wounds. As these dressings absorb exudate, they turn into a gel that keeps the wound bed moist and promotes healing. When exudate is no longer excessive, switch to another type of dressing.

Foam dressings
Foam dressings are spongelike polymer dressings that may be impregnated or coated with other materials. Somewhat absorptive, they may be adherent. These dressings promote moist wound healing and are useful when a nonadherent surface is desired.

Hydrogel dressings
Water-based and nonadherent, hydrogel dressings are polymer-based dressings that have some absorptive properties. They're available as a gel in a tube, as flexible sheets, and as saturated gauze packing strips. They may have a cooling effect, which eases pain, and are used when the wound needs moisture.

age, pull the release paper from the adherent side of the dressing, and apply the dressing to the wound. Hold the dressing in place with your hand (the warmth will mold the dressing to the skin).

Smooth operator

- As you apply the dressing, carefully smooth out wrinkles and avoid stretching the dressing.
- If the dressing's edges need to be secured with tape, apply a skin sealant to the intact skin around the wound. After the area dries, tape the dressing to the skin. The sealant protects the skin from tape burns and skin stripping and promotes tape adherence. Avoid using tension or pressure when applying the tape.
- Remove your gloves and discard them in the impervious plastic trash bag. Dispose of refuse according to facility policy, and wash your hands.

Carefully smooth out wrinkles as you apply the dressing to minimize irritation.

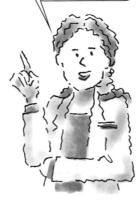

• Change a hydrocolloid dressing every 2 to 7 days as necessary; change it immediately if the patient complains of pain, the dressing no longer adheres, or leakage occurs.

Applying a transparent dressing

• Clean and dry the wound as described above.
• Select a dressing to overlap the wound by 1″ to 2″ (2.5 to 5 cm).
• Gently lay the dressing over the wound; avoid wrinkling the dressing. To prevent shearing force, don't stretch the dressing over the wound. Press firmly on the edges of the dressing to promote adherence. Although this type of dressing is self-adhesive, you may have to tape the edges to prevent them from curling.
• Change the dressing every 3 to 5 days, depending on the amount of drainage. If the seal is no longer secure or if accumulated tissue fluid extends beyond the edges of the wound and onto the surrounding skin, change the dressing.

Applying an alginate dressing

• Apply the alginate dressing to the wound surface. Cover the area with a secondary dressing (such as gauze pads or transparent film) as ordered. Secure the dressing with tape or elastic netting.
• If the wound is draining heavily, change the dressing once or twice daily for the first 3 to 5 days. As drainage decreases, change the dressing less frequently — every 2 to 4 days or as ordered. When the drainage stops or the wound bed looks dry, stop using alginate dressing.

Applying a foam dressing

• Gently lay the foam dressing over the wound.
• Use tape, elastic netting, or gauze to hold the dressing in place.
• Change the dressing when the foam no longer absorbs the exudate.

Applying a hydrogel dressing

• Apply a moderate amount of gel to the wound bed.
• Cover the area with a secondary dressing (gauze, transparent film, or foam).
• Change the dressing daily or as needed to keep the wound bed moist.
• If the hydrogel dressing you select comes in sheet form, cut the dressing to overlap the wound by 1″; then apply as you would a hydrocolloid dressing.
• Hydrogel dressings also come in a prepackaged, saturated gauze for wounds with cavities that require "dead space" to be filled. Follow the manufacturer's directions.

Practice pointers

• Be aware that infection may cause foul-smelling drainage, persistent pain, severe erythema, induration, and elevated skin and body temperatures. Advancing infection or cellulitis can lead to septicemia. Severe erythema may signal worsening cellulitis, which means the offending organisms have invaded the tissue and are no longer localized.

Wound irrigation

Irrigation cleans tissues and flushes cell debris and drainage from an open wound. It also helps prevent premature surface healing over an abscess pocket or infected tract.

After irrigation, pack open wounds to absorb additional drainage. Always follow the standard precaution guidelines of the Centers for Disease Control and Prevention (CDC).

> Irrigation cleans tissues and flushes away cell debris from an open wound.

What you need

Waterproof trash bag ✿ linen-saver pad ✿ emesis basin ✿ clean gloves ✿ sterile gloves, if indicated per facility policy ✿ goggles ✿ gown, if indicated ✿ prescribed irrigant such as sterile normal saline solution ✿ sterile water or normal saline solution ✿ soft rubber or plastic catheter ✿ sterile container ✿ materials as needed for wound care ✿ sterile irrigation and dressing set ✿ commercial wound cleaner ✿ 35-ml piston syringe with 19G needle or catheter ✿ skin protectant wipe (skin sealant) or other protective skin barrier

Getting ready

Assemble equipment in the patient's room. Check the expiration date on each sterile package and inspect for tears.

Don't use any solution that has been open longer than 24 hours. As needed, dilute the prescribed irrigant to the correct proportions with sterile water or normal saline solution. Allow the solution to reach room temperature, or warm it to 90° to 95° F (32.2° to 35° C).

Open the waterproof trash bag; place it near the patient's bed. Form a cuff by turning down the top of the trash bag.

How you do it

- Check the doctor's order, assess the patient's condition, and identify allergies. Explain the procedure to the patient, provide privacy, and position the patient correctly for the procedure. Place the linen-saver pad under the patient and place the emesis basin below the wound so that the irrigating solution flows from the wound into the basin.
- Wash your hands, and put on a gown and gloves.
- Remove the soiled dressing; then discard the dressing and gloves in the trash bag.
- Establish a clean or sterile field with all the equipment and supplies you'll need for wound irrigation and dressing. Pour the prescribed amount of irrigating solution into a clean or sterile container. Put on a new pair of clean gloves and a gown and goggles, if indicated.

From clean to dirty

- Fill the syringe with the irrigating solution and connect the catheter to the syringe. Gently instill a slow, steady stream of solution into the wound until the syringe empties. (See *Irrigating a deep wound.*) Make sure the solution flows from the clean to the dirty area of the wound to prevent contamination of clean tissue by exudate. Also make sure the solution reaches all areas of the wound.
- Refill the syringe, reconnect it to the catheter, and repeat the irrigation. Continue to irrigate the wound until you've administered the prescribed amount of solution or until the solution returns clear. Note the amount of solution administered. Then remove and discard the catheter and syringe in the waterproof trash bag. (See *Wound irrigation tips*, page 62.)

Positioned for success

- Keep the patient positioned to allow further wound drainage into the basin.
- Clean the area around the wound with normal saline solution and pat dry with gauze; wipe intact surrounding skin with a skin protectant wipe and allow it to dry.
- Pack the wound lightly and loosely if ordered, and apply a dressing.
- Remove and discard your gloves and gown.
- Make sure the patient is comfortable.
- Dispose of drainage, solutions, trash bag, and soiled equipment and supplies according to facility policy and CDC guidelines.

> If you aren't careful during irrigation, my pathogenic friends and I will run rampant.

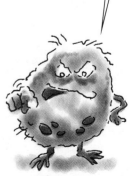

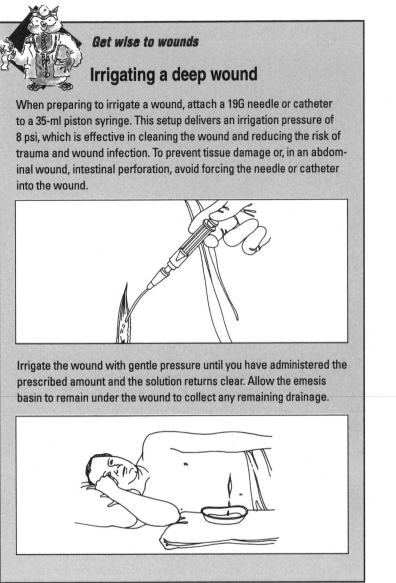

Get wise to wounds

Irrigating a deep wound

When preparing to irrigate a wound, attach a 19G needle or catheter to a 35-ml piston syringe. This setup delivers an irrigation pressure of 8 psi, which is effective in cleaning the wound and reducing the risk of trauma and wound infection. To prevent tissue damage or, in an abdominal wound, intestinal perforation, avoid forcing the needle or catheter into the wound.

Irrigate the wound with gentle pressure until you have administered the prescribed amount and the solution returns clear. Allow the emesis basin to remain under the wound to collect any remaining drainage.

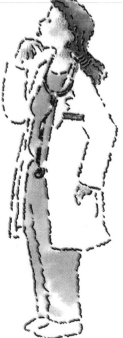

Practice pointers

• Try to coordinate wound irrigation with the doctor's visit so that he can inspect the wound.

• Irrigate with a bulb syringe if the wound is small or not particularly deep or if a piston syringe is unavailable. However, use a bulb syringe cautiously because this type of syringe doesn't deliver enough pressure to adequately clean the wound.

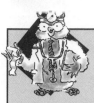

Get wise to wounds

Wound irrigation tips

How can you avoid mess or spillage when irrigating a wound in a hard-to-reach location? Here are some tips you can follow.

Limb wounds

An arm or leg wound may be soaked in a large vessel of warm irrigating fluid, such as water, normal saline solution, or an appropriate antiseptic. An agitator can help dislodge bacteria and loosen debris.

If possible, rinse the wound several times and carefully dispose of the contaminated liquid. Reserve the equipment you used for that particular patient. Dry and store it after soaking it in disinfectant.

Trunk or thigh wounds

Because they're difficult to irrigate, trunk or thigh wounds require some ingenuity. One device uses Stomahesive and a plastic irrigating chamber applied over the wound. (Run warm solution through an infusion set and collect it in a drainage bag.)

A syringe irrigation is another alternative. Where possible, direct the flow at right angles to the wound and allow the fluid to drain by gravity. Doing so requires careful positioning of the patient, either in bed or on a chair. The patient may need analgesia during the treatment.

If irrigation isn't possible, you'll have to swab clean the wound, which is time-consuming. Swab away exudate before using antiseptic or saline solution to clean the wound (taking care not to push loose debris into the wound). Facility policy permitting, use sharp scissors to snip off loose dead tissue—never pull it off.

Debridement

Debridement of nonviable tissue is the most important factor in wound management. Wound healing can't take place until necrotic tissue is removed. Necrotic tissue may present as moist yellow or gray tissue that's separating from viable tissue. If this moist, necrotic tissue becomes dry, it presents as thick, hard, leathery black eschar. Areas of necrotic tissue may mask underlying fluid collections or abscesses. Although debridement can be painful (especially with burns), it's necessary to prevent infection and promote healing of burns and other wounds.

Types of debridement

Debridement of necrotic tissue may be accomplished by sharp, autolytic, chemical, or mechanical techniques.

Sharp debridement

Sharp debridement, which is categorized as either conservative or surgical, involves removing necrotic tissue from the wound bed with the use of a cutting tool, such as a scalpel, scissors, or a laser. Conservative sharp debridement involves the removal of necrotic tissue only and is usually done by a doctor, a physician assistant, an advanced practice nurse, or another certified wound specialist. Surgical sharp debridement involves the removal of both necrotic and healthy tissue, converting a chronic wound to a clean, acute wound. Surgical sharp debridement is typically beyond the practice of nonphysician providers. Caution should be used when providing either conservative or surgical sharp debridement on patients who have low platelet counts or who are taking anticoagulants.

Eschar-go

Conservative sharp debridement of a wound involves careful prying and cutting of loosened eschar with forceps and scissors to separate it from viable tissue beneath. One of the most painful types of debridement, it may require either topical or systemic analgesic administration.

Because you're more likely to be involved in the process of mechanical debridement and conservative sharp debridement, these procedures are covered here in detail.

In autolytic debridement, moisture-retentive dressings are placed over the wound and necrotic tissue dissolves in the wound fluid.

Autolytic debridement

Autolytic debridement involves the use of moisture-retentive dressings to cover the wound bed. Necrotic tissue is then dissolved through self-digestion of enzymes in the wound fluid. Although autolytic debridement takes longer than other debridement methods, it isn't painful, it's easy to do, and it's appropriate for patients who can't tolerate any other method. If the wound is infected, autolytic debridement isn't the treatment of choice.

Chemical debridement

Chemical debridement with enzymatic agents is a selective method of debridement. Enzymes are applied topically to areas of necrotic tissue only, breaking down necrotic tissue elements. Enzymes digest only necrotic tissue — they don't harm healthy tissue. These agents require specific conditions that vary from product to product. Effectiveness is achieved by carefully following each manufacturer's guidelines. Stop using the enzymes when the wound is clean with red granulation tissue.

Mechanical debridement

Mechanical debridement includes wet-to-dry dressings, irrigation, and hydrotherapy. Wet-to-dry dressings, typically used for wounds with extensive necrotic tissue and minimal drainage, require an appropriate technique and the dressing materials used are critical to the outcome. The nurse or doctor places a wet dressing in contact with the lesion and covers it with an outer layer of bandaging. As the dressing dries, it sticks to the wound. When the dried dressing is removed, the necrotic tissue comes off with it.

Irrigation of a wound with a pressurized antiseptic solution cleans tissue and removes wound debris and excess drainage.

Hydrotherapy—commonly referred to as "tubbing," "tanking," or "whirlpool"—involves immersing the patient in a tank of warm water, with intermittent agitation of the water. It's usually performed on large wounds with a significant amount of nonviable tissue covering the wound surface.

What you need

Ordered pain medication ❋ two pairs of sterile gloves ❋ two gowns or aprons ❋ mask ❋ cap ❋ sterile scissors ❋ sterile forceps ❋ sterile 4″ × 4″ gauze pads ❋ sterile solutions and medications as ordered ❋ hemostatic agent as ordered

Hemorrhage emergency

Also have the following equipment immediately available to control bleeding: needle holder ❋ gut suture with needle.

How you do it

• Explain the procedure to the patient to allay his fears and promote cooperation. Teach him distraction and relaxation techniques, if possible, to minimize his discomfort.
• Provide privacy. Per order, administer an analgesic 20 minutes before debridement begins, or give an I.V. analgesic immediately before the procedure.

Wet-to-dry dressings

- Put on clean nonsterile gloves.
- Slowly and gently remove the old dressing, using saline solution to moisten portions of the dressing that don't easily pull away. Discard the old dressing and gloves in a waterproof trash bag.
- Put on clean gloves.
- Using sterile technique, moisten an open-weave cotton gauze dressing with saline solution and loosely pack it into the wound. Make sure the entire wound surface is lightly covered with moistened gauze.
- Apply an outer dressing and secure it with tape or an adhesive bandage.
- Remove the dressing after it completely dries and becomes adherent to the necrotic tissue (typically in 4 to 6 hours).

Irrigation

- Use sterile technique to instill a slow, steady stream of solution into the wound with an irrigating syringe or catheter. (For more information, see the irrigation procedure earlier in this chapter.)

Hydrotherapy

- Prepare the tub, and obtain the patient's vital signs.
- Assist the patient into the tub.
- After the patient or limb has been immersed in the swirling water for the prescribed amount of time (10 to 20 minutes), put on clean gloves, remove the old dressings, and discard all items in a waterproof trash bag.
- Spray rinse and pat dry the patient before reapplying sterile dressings.

Conservative sharp debridement

- Keep the patient warm. Expose only the area to be debrided to prevent chilling and fluid and electrolyte loss.
- Wash your hands, and put on clean gloves.
- Remove the wound dressings and clean the wound.
- Remove your dirty gloves and change into sterile gloves.
- Lift loosened edges of eschar with sterile forceps. Holding the necrotic tissue taut with the forceps, visualize where to cut. Cut the dead tissue from the wound with the scissors.
- Irrigate the wound.

Slim to none

- Because debridement removes only dead tissue, bleeding should be minimal. If bleeding occurs, apply gentle pressure on the wound with sterile 4″ × 4″ gauze pads. Then apply the hemostatic agent. If bleeding persists, notify the doctor and maintain pressure on the wound. Excessive bleeding or spurting vessels may warrant ligation.

- Perform additional procedures, such as application of topical medications and dressing replacements, as ordered.

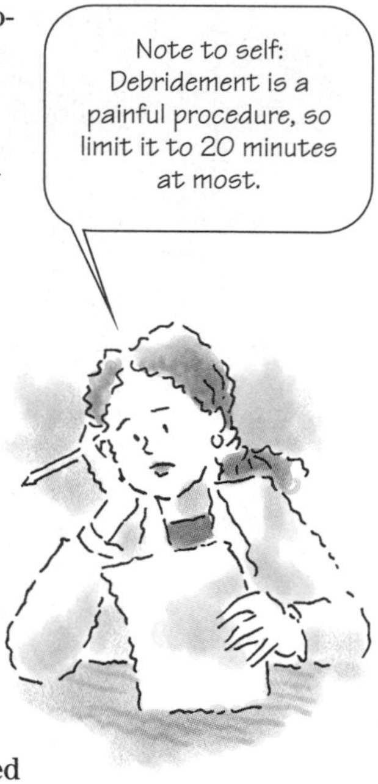
Note to self: Debridement is a painful procedure, so limit it to 20 minutes at most.

Practice pointers

- Acknowledge the patient's discomfort, and provide pain control and emotional support.
- Work quickly — with an assistant if possible — to complete this painful procedure as fast as possible. Try to limit procedure time to 20 minutes. Serial debridement may be necessary to rid the wound of necrotic tissue.

Wound specimen collection

Wound specimen collection involves using a sterile cotton-tipped swab, aspiration with a syringe, or punch tissue biopsy to help identify pathogens.

Because most wounds are colonized with surface bacteria, the swab specimen technique is limited in that it only obtains surface cultures. Needle aspiration of fluid or punch tissue biopsy is recommended for accurate wound culturing. These techniques are performed by doctors, physician assistants, advanced practice nurses, or certified wound specialists.

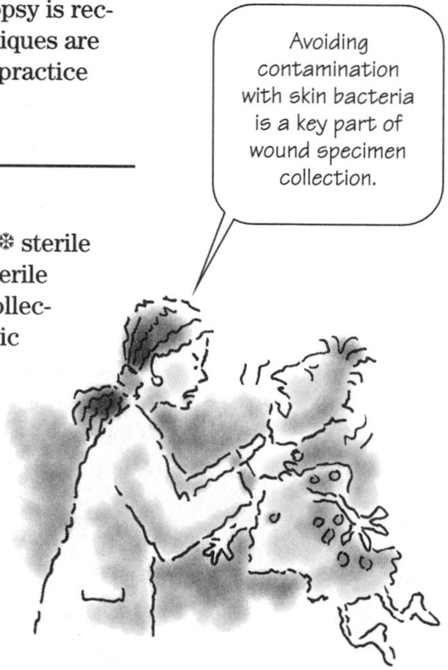
Avoiding contamination with skin bacteria is a key part of wound specimen collection.

What you need

Sterile gloves ❉ alcohol pads or povidone-iodine pads ❉ sterile swabs ❉ sterile 10-ml syringe ❉ sterile 21G needle ❉ sterile culture tube with transport medium (or commercial collection kit for aerobic culture) ❉ labels ❉ special anaerobic culture tube containing carbon dioxide or nitrogen ❉ fresh dressings for the wound ❉ laboratory request form ❉ patient labels

Optional

Rubber stopper for needle

How you do it

- Provide privacy and explain the procedure to the patient.
- Wash your hands, prepare a sterile field, and put on sterile gloves.
- Remove the dressing to expose the wound. Dispose of the soiled dressings properly.
- Clean the wound well.
- Inspect the wound, noting the color, amount, and odor of drainage and presence of necrotic debris.
- Clean the area around the wound with an alcohol pad or a povidone-iodine pad to reduce the risk of contaminating the specimen with skin bacteria. Then allow the area to dry.

Aerobic culture

- Compress the edges of the wound to elicit new drainage.
- Rotate a sterile cotton-tipped swab on the sides and base of the wound bed. If the wound is dry, dip the swab into the transport medium to moisten the tip before swabbing the base of the wound.
- Remove the swab from the wound, and immediately place it in the aerobic culture tube.
- Label the culture tube and send the tube to the laboratory immediately with a completed laboratory request form.
- Never collect exudate from the skin and then insert the same swab into the wound; this could contaminate the wound with skin bacteria.

Anaerobic culture

- Obtain a wound fluid sample as described above. Immediately place it in the anaerobic culture tube (see *Anaerobic specimen collector*, page 68).
- Alternatively, insert a sterile 10-ml syringe, without a needle, into the wound, and aspirate 1 to 5 ml of exudate into the syringe. Then attach the 21G needle to the syringe, and immediately inject the aspirate into the anaerobic culture tube.
- If an anaerobic culture tube is unavailable, obtain a rubber stopper, attach the needle to the syringe, and gently push all the air out of the syringe by pressing on the plunger. Stick the needle tip into the rubber stopper, remove and discard your gloves, and send the syringe of aspirate to the laboratory immediately with a completed laboratory request form.

Anaerobic specimen collector

Because most anaerobes die when exposed to oxygen, they must be transported in tubes filled with carbon dioxide or nitrogen. The anaerobic specimen collector shown here includes a tube filled with carbon dioxide, a small inner tube, and a swab attached to a plastic plunger.

Before specimen collection, the small inner tube containing the swab is held in place with the rubber stopper (as shown below left). After collecting the specimen, quickly replace the swab in the inner tube and depress the plunger to separate the inner tube from the stopper (as shown below right), forcing it into the larger tube and exposing the specimen to a carbon dioxide-rich environment.

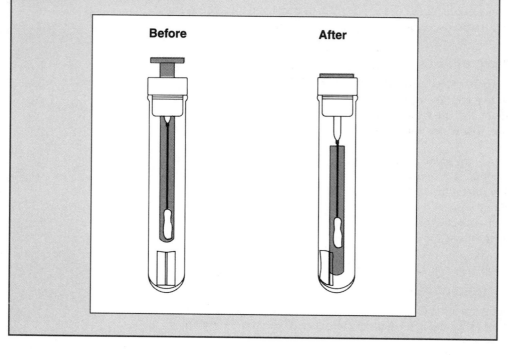

Before   **After**

Practice pointers

- Note recent antibiotic therapy on the laboratory request form.
- Although you would normally clean the area around a wound to prevent contamination by normal skin flora, don't clean a perineal wound with alcohol because this could irritate sensitive tissues. Also, make sure that antiseptic doesn't enter the wound.

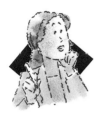

Quick quiz

1. Because mechanical debridement is painful, the procedure should be limited to:

    A.   5 minutes.

    B.   10 minutes.

    C.   20 minutes.

    D.   25 minutes.

Answer: C. Debridement should be done for no more than 20 minutes. If needed, the procedure can be repeated to completely remove the necrotic tissue.

2. To irrigate a wound, direct the flow of irrigant:

    A.   toward the wound.

    B.   away from the wound.

    C.   toward the center of the wound.

    D.   to pool inside of the wound.

Answer: B. Direct flow away from the wound to prevent contamination.

3. The most commonly used cleaning agent is:

    A.   normal saline solution.

    B.   hydrogen peroxide.

    C.   povidone-iodine solution.

    D.   sodium hypochlorite.

Answer: A. Sterile normal saline solution is most commonly used because it provides a moist environment, promotes granulation tissue formation, and causes minimal fluid shifts in healthy adults.

4. Which type of dressing wouldn't be appropriate for a wound with excessive drainage?

    A.   Gauze dressing

    B.   Transparent film dressing

    C.   Alginate dressing

    D.   Hydrocolloid dressing

Answer: B. Because a transparent dressing can't absorb drainage, it should be used only for wounds with minimal drainage.

5. Which methods of wound culturing are most accurate for determining infection?

    A.   Swab technique and needle aspiration

    B.   Swab technique and punch tissue biopsy

    C.   Needle aspiration and punch tissue biopsy

    D.   Aerobic and anaerobic swab techniques

Answer: C. Because the surface of most wounds is normally colonized with bacteria, swab cultures may not be accurate. Needle aspiration and punch tissue biopsy provide the most reliable information.

Scoring

☆☆☆   If you answered all five questions correctly, yippee! Culturally speaking, you're quite a specimen.

☆☆   If you answered three or four questions correctly, great job! You really cleaned up in the area of basic wound care procedures.

☆   If you answered fewer than three questions correctly, don't despair! Order a milkshake to irrigate your system and then review the chapter again.

4

Acute wounds

Just the facts

In this chapter, you'll learn:

♦ types of acute wounds, including those caused by surgery, trauma, and burns

♦ assessment factors for each type of acute wound

♦ the way skin grafts are used to repair defects caused by acute wounds.

A look at acute wounds

As you know, three aspects are used to classify wounds and determine wound severity: age, depth, and color. Wound age is typically described as acute or chronic. Seems simple enough until you ask, "At what point does an acute wound become a chronic wound?" Time alone is not the distinguishing factor. Progress toward complete healing is also a component. Therefore, an acute wound is better characterized by these criteria:
• it's a new or relatively new wound
• it occurred suddenly (as opposed to developing over time)
• healing is progressing in a timely and predictable manner.

Intent or accident?

Acute wounds can occur by intention or trauma. A surgical incision is an example of an acute wound that's caused intentionally. Traumatic wounds can range from simple to severe. We'll take a close look at each category in this chapter. Burns are a category of traumatic wound that have a unique set of causes, potential complications, and treatment options, so we'll look at them separately.

Regardless of the cause, caring for a patient with an acute wound focuses on restoring normal anatomic structure, physiologic function, and appearance to the wound area.

> Don't wait around for time to determine if your patient's wound is acute or chronic. Use these assessment criteria.

Surgical wounds

An acute surgical wound is a healthy and uncomplicated break in the skin's continuity resulting from surgery. In an otherwise healthy individual, this type of wound responds well to postoperative care and heals without incident.

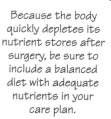

Looks like we're both at risk. Skin variations related to age can play an important role in wound healing.

Factors that affect healing

Several factors can greatly affect the course of postoperative healing. These include the patient's age, nutritional status, general health before surgery, and oxygenation status.

Age

Age is an important factor in the healing process, especially for pediatric patients and older adults. In a premature infant, for example, the immune system and other body systems aren't fully developed and, thus, he's at greater risk for infection before, during, and after surgery. Sterile technique is a critical component of care for such patients.

Prolonged repair

At the other end of the age continuum, older adults commonly have a harder time healing after surgery due to skin changes. As a person ages, skin becomes thinner and less elastic. Populations of the cells that repair tissues and fight infection decline, and the skin's vascular system is less robust. As a result, surgical wounds in older patients heal more slowly, increasing the risk of infection.

Nutrition

Proper nutrition is crucial for the body to heal itself effectively. During your assessment, it's imperative for you to identify nutritional problems early and to develop a plan that addresses deficits.

After surgery, the body quickly depletes its stores of nutrients and even an otherwise healthy patient can become malnourished if diet is ignored. The care plan must include a diet with adequate nutrients to maintain homeostasis and create an optimum environment for wound healing.

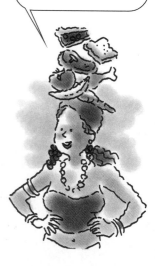

Because the body quickly depletes its nutrient stores after surgery, be sure to include a balanced diet with adequate nutrients in your care plan.

Adipose poses problems

A patient who's overweight has an additional problem. Adipose tissue lacks the extensive vascular supply present in skin. As the amount of adipose tissue increases, blood flow to the skin decreases. This reduces the amount of oxygen and nutrients reaching the area of the wound and impedes healing.

Illness or infection

In most cases, a preexisting illness or infection delays or complicates healing after surgery. Unfortunately, it isn't always possible to delay surgery while an underlying condition resolves itself. In these cases, the care plan must include measures that minimize the impact of the preexisting condition on the healing process. For example:

• Disorders that impede blood flow, such as coronary artery disease, peripheral vascular disease, and hypertension, can cause problems by reducing the flow of blood reaching the incision site. A patient with one of these conditions requires a care plan that includes interventions to improve circulation.

• Cancer may necessitate more aggressive pain management or a care plan that includes management of such symptoms as nausea and vomiting.

• Diabetes mellitus impedes healing in many ways and increases the patient's risk of infection. Diabetic neuropathy (inflammation and degeneration of peripheral nerves), if present, may interfere with vasodilation and, consequently, circulation in the area of the incision.

• Immunosuppression resulting from either a disease or drug therapy (corticosteroids, chemotherapy) may impair the inflammatory response, delaying wound healing and increasing the patient's risk of infection. Care should focus on keeping the wound clean and protecting it from trauma.

> Some drugs cause immunosuppression, which delays wound healing and increases the patient's risk of infection.

Stopping on red

A preexisting infection can also delay or impair healing. Signs of wound infection include:

• increased exudate
• purulent (pus-containing) exudate
• erythema (reddened tissue) around the wound
• warmer skin temperature at or around the wound
• new or increased pain
• general malaise
• fever

• high white blood cell count.

All open wounds are colonized with surface bacteria, but infected wounds are slow to heal and may become dehisced or eviscerated.

Oxygenation status

During healing, neutrophils require oxygen to produce the hydrogen peroxide they use to kill pathogens, and fibroblasts require oxygen for collagen proliferation. Therefore, adequate oxygenation is critical to the healing process. Any condition that impedes overall oxygenation or the amount of oxygen reaching the wound — atherosclerosis, for example — slows the healing process.

Assessment and care

Proper care during healing varies depending on the method of wound closure used, the development of the healing ridge, and the type of dressing ordered. The patient's ability to properly perform wound care after discharge also affects healing.

Wound closure

The surgeon determines the appropriate method of wound closure based on the wound's severity; in most cases, sutures are used.

Sew...a needle pulling thread

In suturing, a natural or synthetic thread is used to stitch the wound closed. (See *Suture materials and methods*.)

Sutures typically remain in place for 7 to 10 days, provided that healing is progressing as expected. Factors that affect the timing of suture removal include the patient's overall condition; the shape, size, and location of the incision; and whether inflammation, drainage, or infection develops.

Stainless steel solutions

The surgeon may choose to use skin staples or clips as an alternative to sutures if cosmetic results aren't an issue. These closures secure a wound faster than sutures and, because they're made of surgical stainless steel, tissue reaction is minimal. Properly placed staples and clips distribute tension evenly along the suture line, reducing tissue trauma and compression. This promotes healing and minimizes scarring. The surgeon won't use staples or clips if less than 5 mm of tissue exists between the staple and any underlying bone, vessel, or organ.

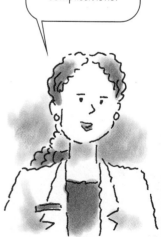

Sutures typically remain in place for 7 to 10 days, as long as there aren't any complications.

Suture materials and methods

When closing a surgical wound, the choice of suture material varies according to the suturing method.

Materials

Nonabsorbable sutures are used to close the skin surface. They provide strength and immobility and minimize tissue irritation. Nonabsorbable suture materials include silk, cotton, stainless steel, and Dacron.

When suture removal is undesirable—for example, sutures in an underlying tissue layer—the surgeon chooses an *absorbable suture.* Absorbable suture materials include:
• chromic catgut—a natural catgut treated with chromium trioxide to improve strength and prolong absorption time
• plain catgut—a material that's absorbed faster and is more likely to cause irritation than chromic catgut
• synthetic materials—materials such as polyglycolic acid that are replacing catgut because they're stronger, more durable, and less irritating.

Methods

The most common suture methods include mattress continuous suture, plain continuous suture, mattress interrupted suture, plain interrupted suture, and blanket continuous suture. These methods are described here.

Mattress continuous suture

Mattress continuous suture is a series of connected mattress stitches with a knot at the beginning and end.

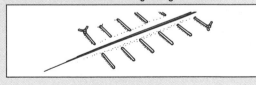

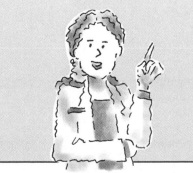

Plain continuous suture

Also called a continuous running suture, a plain continuous suture is a series of connected stitches. The thread is knotted at the beginning and at the end of the suture.

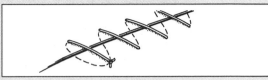

Mattress interrupted suture

Mattress interrupted suture is a series of independent stitches, similar to plain interrupted suture. However, in this suture, both threads cross beneath the suture line, leaving only a small portion of suture exposed on each side of the wound.

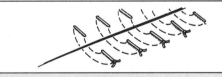

Plain interrupted suture

In a plain interrupted suture, the doctor sews individual sutures, each with a separate piece of thread. Half of the thread length crosses under the suture line; the other half crosses above the skin surface.

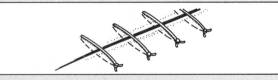

Blanket continuous suture

Blanket continuous suture is a series of looped stitches with a knot at the beginning and end of the series.

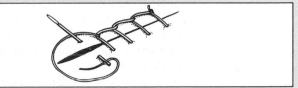

Types of adhesive skin closures

The two most common types of adhesive skin closures are Steri-Strips and butterfly closures.

Steri-Strips
Steri-Strips, thin strips of sterile, nonwoven tape, are a primary means of holding a wound closed after suture removal.

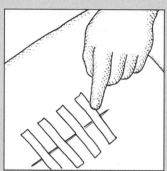

Butterfly closures
Butterfly closures have two sterile, waterproof adhesive strips connected by a narrow, nonadhesive "bridge." These strips are used to hold small wounds closed to promote healing after suture removal.

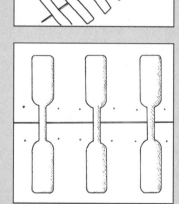

Stick with me!

Smaller wounds with little drainage can be closed with adhesive skin closures, such as Steri-Strips or butterfly closures. As with staples and clips, these closures cause little tissue reaction. Adhesive closures can be used after suture or staple removal to provide ongoing support for a healing incision. (See *Types of adhesive skin closures*.)

The healing ridge

To properly assess healing, it's important to understand how the healing ridge develops in an incision after surgery. The healing ridge is a buildup of collagen fibers that begins to form during the inflammatory phase of wound healing and peaks during the proliferation phase (approximately days 5 to 9). You can feel this ridge as you gently palpate the skin on each side of the wound. The healing ridge is a sign that healing is progressing. If you can't feel this ridge, healing isn't progressing as expected and further assessment is required. In cases where the ridge fails to develop, mechanical strain on the wound is most likely at fault.

Dressings

The incision dressing shields the wound against pathogens and protects the skin surface from irritating drainage. The dressing is the primary aspect of wound management for surgical wounds; therefore, choosing the right type is important.

Typically, lightly exuding wounds with drains and wounds with minimal purulent drainage require only packing and a gauze dressing. A wound with copious, excoriating drainage requires an absorbent dressing, such as an alginate, or pouching to contain the drainage and protect the surrounding skin. (See *Pouching a wound*, page 78.)

When dressing a surgical wound, use sterile technique and sterile supplies to prevent contamination. Change the dressing as often as needed to absorb drainage and keep the surrounding skin dry. However, remember that a wound heals best at body temperature. Changing the dressing lowers the temperature at the wound site and healing slows until the site returns to normal body temperature.

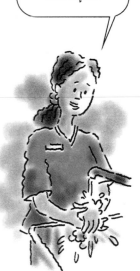

Start patient teaching with the basics — asepsis and hand-washing techniques.

Patient education

Patient education is an important care plan component for patients with surgical wounds. By the time he's discharged, the patient needs to understand — and demonstrate — the ability to perform proper wound care. Start with an assessment of the patient's knowledge. Then begin teaching with a discussion of basic asepsis and hand-washing techniques. The balance of your teaching depends on the type of surgery, the type of dressing, and the location of the wound. (See *Teaching about surgical wound care*, page 79.)

Potential complications

Surgery results in a controlled form of acute wound. The patient's environment, the type and severity of the wound, and preoperative and postoperative care are all under the control of members of the health care team. Consequently, most surgical wounds heal without incident. Some complications that might arise, however, include wound infection, hemorrhage, and wound dehiscence and evisceration.

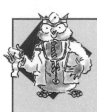

Get wise to wounds

Pouching a wound

If your patient's wound is draining heavily or if drainage may damage surrounding skin, you need to apply a pouch. Here's how:
• Measure the wound. Cut an opening ⅜" larger than the wound in the facing of the collection pouch (see photo below).

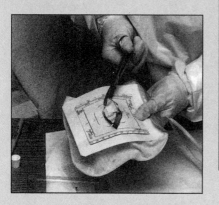

• Apply a skin protectant as needed. (Some protectants are incorporated into the collection pouch system and also provide adhesion.)

• Be sure to close the drainage port at the bottom of the pouch to prevent leaks. Then gently press the contoured pouch opening around the wound, starting at the lower edge, to catch any drainage (see photo below).

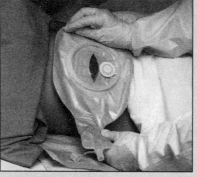

• To empty the pouch, put on gloves, a face shield or mask, and eye protection. Insert the lower portion of the pouch into a graduated biohazard container and open the drainage port (see photo top right). Note the color, consistency, odor, and amount of fluid. If ordered, obtain a culture specimen and send it to

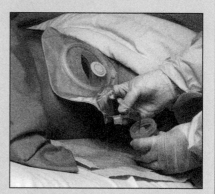

the laboratory immediately. Always follow Centers for Disease Control and Prevention standard precautions when handling infectious drainage.
• Use a gauze pad to wipe the bottom of the pouch and the drainage port. This prevents skin irritation or possible odor from any residual drainage. Reseal the port.
• Change the pouch only if it leaks or fails to adhere. More frequent changes are unnecessary and can irritate the patient's skin.

Wound infection

Wound infection is the most common wound complication as well as the second most common nosocomial infection (infection contracted during hospitalization). Preventing wound infection requires meticulous attention to sterile technique when caring for the wound.

> ## Teaching about surgical wound care
>
> Surgical patients need to know the ways they can promote healing and prevent infection. Be sure to discuss:
> - signs and symptoms of wound infection that should be reported to the doctor immediately, such as increased tenderness, deep or increased pain at the wound site, fever, or edema (especially if it occurs between postoperative days 3 and 5)
> - the way to obtain an accurate temperature reading
> - proper wound care, such as the importance of keeping the incision clean and dry; proper hand-washing technique; and the supplies and methods used to clean the wound
> - wound dressings, including the type, proper application methods, and places to obtain them
> - types and levels of permissible activity, such as when the patient may shower or bathe, any restrictions on lifting (if applicable), and when the patient can expect to return to work
> - follow-up appointments.

Mean to intervene

For a surgical patient, wound infection is a significant and serious event requiring prompt intervention. Interventions typically ordered in cases of postoperative infection include:
- obtaining a wound culture and sensitivity test
- administering antibiotics
- irrigating the wound
- dressing the wound and packing it, if necessary
- monitoring wound drainage.

Hemorrhage

Hemorrhage may occur from damage to blood vessels. In the postoperative patient, it may happen in either internal or external sites:
- The most common locations of significant internal hemorrhages are the posterior nasal passages, pulmonary vessels, spleen, liver, stomach, and uterus. Hemorrhage may also occur at the site of a large artery injury or aneurysm. Hemorrhage in one of these areas significantly reduces the volume of circulating blood and precipitates hypovolemia. Nursing interventions include administering I.V. fluids to increase blood pressure and urine output and helping determine the source of bleeding.

• If the hemorrhage originates externally—for example, from the wound itself or from damage to the fragile, newly developed blood vessels—place pressure or a pressure dressing on the site of the bleeding and notify the doctor for specific treatment orders.

Wound dehiscence and evisceration

Dehiscence is most likely to occur when collagen fibers aren't mature enough to hold the incision closed without sutures. The first sign of dehiscence may be an abscess or a gush of serosanguinous fluid from the wound or a report from the patient of a "popping" sensation after coughing or retching. Complete dehiscence leads to evisceration, in which underlying tissues protrude through the wound opening. Abdominal wounds are more likely to dehisce and eviscerate than thoracic wounds.

An ounce of prevention

To prevent wound dehiscence and evisceration, teach the patient to support the incision with a pillow or cushion before he changes position, coughs, or sneezes.

If dehiscence occurs, take these steps:
• Stay with the patient; keep him still and have a colleague notify the doctor.
• If the patient has an abdominal wound, help him into low Fowler's position, with knees bent to reduce abdominal tension.
• If evisceration is evident, cover extruding tissues with warm, sterile normal saline soaks.

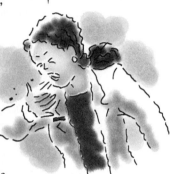

Achoo! To help prevent dehiscence and evisceration, teach your patient to support the incision with a pillow or cushion before he changes position, coughs, or sneezes.

Traumatic wounds

A traumatic wound is a sudden, unplanned injury to the skin that can range from minor (such as a skinned knee) to severe (such as a gunshot wound). This category of wounds includes abrasions, lacerations, skin tears, bites, and penetrating trauma wounds.

Abrasions

An abrasion occurs when a mechanical force, such as friction or shearing, scrapes away a partial thickness of the skin. Unless an unusually large amount of skin is involved or an infection develops, an abrasion is one of the least complicated traumatic wounds.

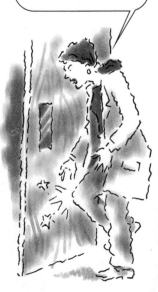

It may not seem too traumatic, but even a minor abrasion such as a skinned knee is considered a traumatic wound.

Preventing skin tears

As aging occurs, the skin becomes more prone to skin tear injuries. With a little effort and education, you can substantially reduce a patient's risk. Prevent skin tears by:

• using proper lifting, positioning, transferring, and turning techniques to reduce or eliminate friction or shear

• padding support surfaces where risk is greatest, such as bed rails and limb supports on a wheelchair

• using pillows or cushions to support the patient's arms and legs

• telling the patient to add protection by wearing long-sleeved shirts and long pants, as weather permits

• using nonadhering dressings or those with minimal adherent, such as paper tape, and to use a skin barrier wipe before applying dressings

• removing tape cautiously using the push-pull technique

• using wraps, such as a stockinette or soft gauze, to protect areas of skin where the risk of tearing is high

• telling the patient to avoid sudden or brusque movements that can pull the skin and possibly cause a skin tear

• applying skin lotion twice per day to areas at risk.

Lacerations

A laceration is a tear in the skin that's caused by a sharp object, such as metal, glass, or wood. It can also be caused by trauma that produces high shearing force. A laceration has jagged, irregular edges and its severity depends on its cause, size, depth, and location.

Skin tears

A skin tear is a specific type of laceration that most often affects older adults. In a skin tear, friction alone — or shearing force plus friction — separate layers of skin. A partial-thickness wound occurs if the epidermis separates from the dermis; a full-thickness wound occurs if the epidermis and dermis separate from underlying tissue. This type of injury may be preventable through careful handling by members of the health care team. (See *Preventing skin tears.*)

Bites

When assessing a bite wound, it's important to quickly discover the bite's source — cat, dog, bat, snake, spider, human? This helps the health care team determine which bacteria or toxins may be present and the likely type of tissue trauma.

Hannibal the cannibal?

For example, a human bite can cause a puncture wound and introduce any one of the innumerable organisms present in the human mouth into the wound. *Staphylococcus aureus* and streptococci are two such organisms that can be transmitted to the wound or into the victim's bloodstream. Other serious diseases that can be transmitted in this way include human immunodeficiency virus infection, hepatitis B, hepatitis C, syphilis, and tuberculosis. Some evidence suggests that a human bite can also cause necrotizing fasciitis.

Animal house

Be aware that bites from such animals as dogs, cats, and rabbits can cause rabies in addition to possible tissue damage.

A bite from a dog, cat, or rodent can introduce deadly infectious diseases, such as rabies, into the wound. In terms of tissue damage, cats and other smaller mammals do relatively little damage. However, a dog can generate up to 200 psi of pressure when biting and if he shakes his head at the same time, which is usually the case, strong torsional force is brought to bear. Together, these forces can cause a massive amount of tissue damage.

Penetrating trauma wounds

A penetrating trauma wound is a puncture wound. This type of wound may be the result of an accident or a personal attack, as in the case of a stabbing or gunshot wound.

Not so knife

Stab wounds are low-velocity wounds that generally present as classic puncture wounds or lacerations. In some cases, however, they may involve organ damage beneath the site of the wound. X-rays, computed tomography scanning, and magnetic resonance imaging are used to evaluate possible organ damage. If the weapon used is contaminated, the patient is at risk for, and should be treated for, local infection, sepsis, and tetanus.

Bullet wound blues

A gunshot wound is a high-velocity wound. Factors that affect the severity of tissue damage include the caliber of the weapon, the velocity of the projectile, and the patient's position at the time of injury.

In most cases, a small-caliber weapon firing a relatively low-velocity projectile creates a small, clean punctuate lesion with little or no bleeding. If the projectile is no longer in the patient's body, treat this lesion as you would any other open wound.

A large-caliber, relatively high-velocity projectile typically causes massive tissue destruction, a large gaping wound, profuse bleeding and wound contamination. In this case, the patient usually requires immediate surgical intervention. After surgery, treat the wound as a surgical wound.

Assessment and care

Time is critical when caring for a patient with a traumatic wound. First, assess airway, breathing, and circulation (ABCs). Although focusing first on the injury itself may seem natural, a patent airway and pumping heart take priority.

Next, turn your attention to the wound. Control bleeding by applying firm, direct pressure and elevate the patient's extremities. If bleeding continues, you may need to compress a pressure point above the wound. Then assess the wound's condition. Specific wound management and cleaning depend on the type of wound and degree of contamination. (See *Caring for a traumatic wound*, page 84.)

Special considerations

In caring for a patient with a traumatic wound, pay particular attention to the following aspects of care:
• When irrigating the wound, avoid using more than 8 psi of pressure. High-pressure irrigation can seriously interfere with healing by destroying cells and forcing bacteria into the tissue.
• When cleaning the wound, use sterile normal saline solution to remove debris. Never instill hydrogen peroxide into a deep wound — the evolving gases can cause an embolism.

Prohibition

• Avoid using alcohol to clean a traumatic wound. It's painful for the patient and it dehydrates tissue. Similarly, avoid cleaning with antiseptics because they can impede healing.
• Never use a cotton ball or a cotton-filled gauze pad to clean a wound because cotton fibers left in the wound may cause contamination or a foreign body reaction.
• If the doctor plans to debride the wound to remove dead tissue and reduce the risk of infection and scarring, pack the wound with gauze pads soaked in normal saline solution until it's time for the procedure.
• Monitor closely for signs of developing infection, such as warm red skin or purulent discharge from the wound. Infection in a trau-

Get wise to wounds

Caring for a traumatic wound

When treating a patient with a traumatic wound, always begin by assessing the ABCs: airway, breathing, and circulation. Move on to the wound itself only after ABCs are stable. Here are the basic steps to follow in caring for each type of traumatic wound.

Abrasion
• Flush the area of the abrasion with normal saline solution or wound cleaning solution.
• Use a sterile 4″ × 4″ gauze pad moistened with normal saline solution to remove dirt or gravel, and gently rub toward the entry point to work contaminants back out the way they entered.
• If the wound is extremely dirty, you may need to scrub it with a surgical brush. Be as gentle as possible and keep in mind that this is a painful process for your patient.
• Allow a small wound to dry and form a scab. Cover larger wounds with a nonadherent pad or petroleum gauze and a light dressing. Apply antibacterial ointment if ordered.

Laceration
• Moisten a sterile 4″ × 4″ gauze pad with normal saline solution or wound cleaning solution. Gently clean the wound, beginning at the center and working out to approximately 2″ (5 cm) beyond the edge of the wound. Whenever the pad becomes soiled, discard it and use a new one. Continue until the wound appears clean.
• If necessary, irrigate the wound using a 50 ml catheter-tip syringe and normal saline solution.
• Assist the doctor in suturing the wound if necessary; apply sterile strips of porous tape if suturing isn't needed.
• Apply antibacterial ointment as ordered to prevent infection.

• Apply a dry sterile dressing over the wound to absorb drainage and help prevent bacterial contamination.

Bite
• Immediately irrigate the wound with copious amounts of normal saline solution. Don't immerse and soak the wound; this may allow bacteria to float back into the tissue.
• Clean the wound with sterile 4″ × 4″ gauze pads and an antiseptic solution such as povidone-iodine.
• Assist with debridement if ordered.
• Apply a loose dressing. If the bite is on an extremity, elevate it to reduce swelling.
• Ask the patient about the animal that bit him to determine whether there's a risk of rabies. Administer rabies and tetanus shots as needed.

Penetrating wound
• If the wound is minor, allow it to bleed for a few minutes before cleaning it. A larger puncture wound may require irrigation.
• Cover the wound with a dry dressing.
• If the wound contains an embedded foreign object, such as a shard of glass or metal, stabilize the object until the doctor can remove it. When the object is removed and bleeding is under control, clean the wound as you would a laceration.

matic wound can delay healing, increase scarring, and trigger systemic infections such as septicemia.
• Inspect the dressings regularly. If edema develops, adjust the dressing to ensure adequate circulation to the area of the wound.

Burns

A burn is an acute wound caused by exposure to thermal extremes, caustic chemicals, electricity, or radiation. The degree of tissue damage depends on the strength of the source and the duration of contact or exposure.

Thermal burns

Thermal burns, the most common type of burn, can result from virtually any misuse or mishandling of fire or a combustible product. Playing with matches, pouring gasoline into a hot lawnmower, and setting off fireworks are some common examples of ways in which burns occur. Thermal burns can also result from kitchen accidents, house or office fires, automobile accidents, or physical abuse. Although less common, exposure to extreme cold can also cause thermal burns.

Chemical burns

Chemical burns most commonly result from contact (skin contact or inhalation) with a caustic agent, such as an acid, an alkali, or a vesicant.

Electrical burns

Electrical burns result from contact with flowing electrical current. Household current, high-voltage transmission lines, and lightning are sources of electrical burns.

Radiation burns

The most common radiation burn is sunburn, which follows excessive exposure to the sun. Almost all other burns due to radiation exposure occur as a result of radiation treatment or in specific industries that use or process radioactive materials.

Assessment

Initial assessment should be conducted as soon as possible after the burn occurs. First, assess ABCs. Then determine the patient's level of consciousness and mobility. After this, assess the burn, including burn size, depth, and severity.

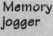

Memory jogger

This alphabetic mnemonic describes the proper sequence for initial assessment of a burn patient:

Airway — Assess the patient's airway; remove any obstruction and treat any obstructive condition.

Breathing — Observe the motion of the patient's chest. Auscultate the depth, rate, and character of the patient's breathing.

Circulation — Palpate the pulse at the carotid artery and then at the distal pulse points in the wrist, posterior tibial area, and foot. Loss of distal pulse may indicate shock or constriction of an extremity.

Disability — Assess the patient's level of consciousness and ability to function before attempting to move or transfer him.

Expose — Remove burned clothing from burned areas of the body and thoroughly examine the skin beneath.

Estimating burn size

Because body surface area (BSA) varies with age, two different methods are used to estimate burn size in adult and pediatric patients.

Rule of Nines

You can quickly estimate the extent of an adult patient's burn by using the Rule of Nines. This method quantifies BSA in multiples of 9, thus the name. To use this method, mentally transfer the burns on your patient to the body charts below. Add the corresponding percentages for each body section burned. Use the total—a rough estimate of burn extent—to calculate initial fluid replacement needs.

Lund and Browder Classification

The Rule of Nines isn't accurate for infants or children because their body shapes, and therefore BSA, differ from those of adults. For example, an infant's head accounts for about 17% of his total BSA, compared with 7% for an adult. Instead, use the Lund and Browder Classification to determine burn size for infants and children.

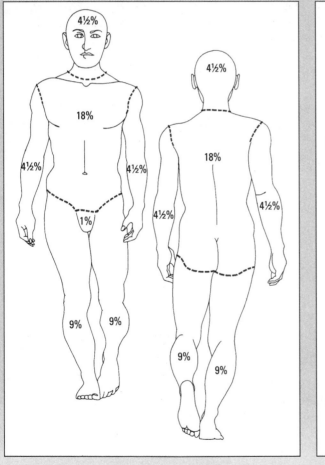

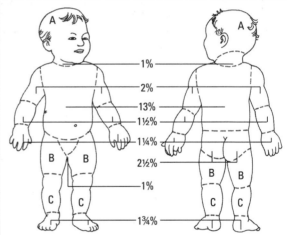

Percentage of burned body surface by age

	At birth	0 to 1 year	1 to 4 years	5 to 9 years	10 to 15 years	Adult
A: Half of head						
	9½%	8½%	6½%	5½%	4½%	3½%
B: Half of one thigh						
	2¾%	3¼%	4%	4¼%	4½%	4¾%
C: Half of one leg						
	2½%	2½%	2¾%	3%	3¼%	3½%

Determining size

Determine burn size as part of your initial assessment. Typically, burn size is expressed as a percentage of total body surface area (BSA). The Rule of Nines and the Lund and Browder Classification are two useful tools for providing reasonably standardized and quick estimates of the percentage of BSA affected. (See *Estimating burn size.*)

Determining depth

During the initial assessment, determine burn depth. A partial-thickness burn involves the epidermis and part of the dermis. A full-thickness burn involves the epidermis, dermis, and subcutaneous tissue.

Four degrees of separation

The traditional method of gauging burn severity classifies burn depth by degree:

first-degree — damage is limited to the epidermis, causing erythema and pain

second-degree — the epidermis and part of the dermis are damaged, producing blisters, mild-to-moderate edema, and pain

third-degree — the epidermis and dermis are damaged; no blisters appear, but white, brown, or black leathery tissue and thrombosed vessels are visible

fourth-degree — damage extends through deeply charred subcutaneous tissue to muscle and bone.

In most instances, damage involves several depths and degrees. (See *Visualizing burn depth,* page 88.)

Determining severity

The severity of a burn is associated with both its size and depth. The three categories of burn severity are major, moderate, and minor.

Major

Major burns meet one or more of these criteria:
• third-degree burns on more than 10% of BSA
• second-degree burns on more than 25% of BSA in adults; more than 20% in children
• burns on the hands, face, feet, or genitalia
• burns complicated by fractures or respiratory damage
• electrical burns
• any burn in a poor-risk patient.

Visualizing burn depth

The most widely used system of classifying burn depth and severity categorizes them by degree. However, it's important to remember that most burns involve tissue damage of different degrees and thicknesses. This illustration may help you visualize burn damage at the various degrees.

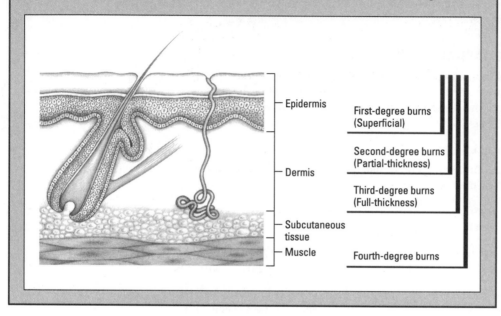

- Epidermis — First-degree burns (Superficial)
- Dermis — Second-degree burns (Partial-thickness)
- Third-degree burns (Full-thickness)
- Subcutaneous tissue
- Muscle — Fourth-degree burns

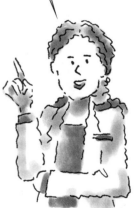

Remember, when determining burn severity, you must take into account not only the size of the wound but also the depth.

Moderate

Moderate burns meet one or more of these criteria:
- third-degree burns on 2% to 10% of BSA
- second-degree burns on 15% to 25% of BSA in adults, 10% to 20% of BSA in children.

Minor

Minor burns meet one or more of these criteria:
- third-degree burns on less than 2% of BSA
- second-degree burns on less than 15% of BSA in adults, less than 10% of BSA in children.

Special assessment considerations

When assessing a burn victim, pay particular attention to factors that affect treatment and healing, including:
- burn location — burns on the face, hands, feet, and genitalia are most serious due to the possible loss of function
- burn configuration — edema due to a circumferential burn (one that goes completely around an extremity) can slow or stop circu-

lation to the extremity; burns on the neck can obstruct the airway; burns on the chest can interfere with normal respiration by inhibiting expansion
- preexisting medical conditions—note disorders that impair peripheral circulation, especially diabetes, peripheral vascular disease, and chronic alcohol abuse
- other injuries sustained at the time of the burn
- patient age—victims under age 4 or over age 60 are at higher risk for complications and, consequently, for a higher mortality rate
- pulmonary injury—inhaling smoke or super-heated air damages lung tissue.

Burn care

Care for a burn patient depends on the type and severity of the burn, the patient's general health before the injury, and whether another injury was sustained concurrent with the burn. In general, treatment seeks to reduce pain; remove dirt, debris, and dead tissue; and provide a dressing that promotes healing. In some cases, treatment includes skin grafting.

Minor to moderate burns

In minor to moderate burns, the first step is to stop the burning process and relieve pain. Remove smoldering clothing and provide pain medication, as ordered. When cleaning the burns, never use hydrogen peroxide or povidone-iodine (or products containing these agents) because they can cause further tissue damage. Cover the burns with dry, sterile towels.

Something to talk about

As soon as the patient's condition stabilizes, and other injuries are ruled out, the doctor may order a narcotic analgesic, such as morphine or meperidine. Be sure to talk to the patient as you work. Emotional support and reassurance are important aspects of care and may reduce the patient's need for analgesia.

Wrapping it up

After the doctor debrides devitalized tissue, if necessary, cover the wound with an antimicrobial and a nonadhesive bulky dressing. If ordered, administer tetanus prophylaxis.

Moderate to major burns

In moderate to major burns, immediately assess the patient's ABCs. Be especially alert for signs of smoke inhalation and pulmonary damage—singed nasal hairs, mucosal burns, changes in the patient's voice, coughing, wheezing, soot in the mouth or nose, or darkened sputum. If necessary, assist with endotracheal intubation and administer 100% oxygen. When the patient's ABCs are stable, take a brief history of the burn and draw blood samples, as ordered, for diagnostic tests.

The next step is to stop residual burning and control bleeding. Remove any smoldering clothing. If material is stuck to the patient's skin, soak it with saline solution before you attempt to remove it. Remove all jewelry and any other constricting items of apparel. Then cover the burns with a clean, dry, sterile bed sheet. (Never cover large burns with saline-soaked dressings because this can drastically lower body temperature).

Solution resolution

Begin I.V. therapy, as ordered, to prevent hypovolemic shock and help maintain cardiac output. A patient with serious burns needs massive fluid replacement—especially during the first 24 hours after the injury. At this juncture, the doctor may order a combination of crystalloids such as lactated Ringer's solution.

What goes in must come out

Closely monitor the patient's intake and output, and check vital signs often. If the patient's limbs are badly burned, measuring blood pressure can be nerve wracking; however, be sure to check blood pressure as required by applying a sterile nonstick pad to the area first. Finally, be prepared to assist in emergency escharotomy if the patient's burns threaten circulation.

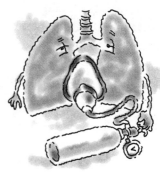

Gasp! I prefer the nonsmoking section. In cases of smoke inhalation, I may need for you to administer 100% oxygen.

Electrical burns

Tissue damage from electrical burns is difficult to assess because internal damage along the conduction pathway is commonly greater than the surface burn indicates. If possible, determine the voltage involved. This information helps the health care team assess possible internal damage more accurately.

Keep in mind that current passing through the body can induce ventricular fibrillation, cardiac arrest, or respiratory arrest—all life-threatening conditions requiring immediate intervention. (See *Electric shock.*)

Chemical burns

When treating a patient with a chemical burn, begin by irrigating the wound with plenty of sterile water or normal saline solution. Using a weak base, such as sodium bicarbonate, to neutralize an acid spilled on the skin or mucous membranes is controversial,

Electric shock

When electric current passes through the body, the damage it does depends on the:
• intensity of the current (measured in amperes)
• resistance of the tissues it passes through
• kind of current (alternating current, direct current, or a combination of both)
• frequency and duration of the flow of current.
   Electric current can cause injury in three ways:
• true electrical injury caused by current that passes through the body
• arc or flash burns caused by current that doesn't pass through the body
• thermal surface burns caused by associated heat and flames.
   Prognosis depends on:
• site of the injury
• extent of damage
• patient's general health prior to the injury
• speed and adequacy of treatment.

particularly during the emergency phase, because the neutralizing agent can generate more heat, causing additional tissue damage.

If the patient's eyes are involved, flush them with plenty of water or saline solution for at least 30 minutes. If it's an alkaline burn, irrigate until the pH of the cul-de-sacs returns to 7.0. Then have the patient close his eyes and cover them with dry, sterile dressings. Arrange for an ophthalmologic examination. Finally, note the type of chemical involved and the presence of any noxious fumes.

If the patient is to be transferred to a burn care unit soon after the accident, wrap him first in a sterile sheet and then a blanket for warmth and elevate the burned extremity to minimize edema.

Skin grafting

Skin grafting may be necessary to repair defects caused by burns, trauma, or surgery. Depending on the graft's complexity, the procedure may be performed under local or general anesthesia and, in some cases, may be performed as an outpatient procedure. (For information on temporary skin grafts, see *Biological dressings*, page 92.)

The surgeon may choose skin grafting as the preferred treatment option if:
• primary closure isn't possible or cosmetically acceptable

Dress for success

Biological dressings

Biological dressings function much like skin grafts, preventing infection and fluid loss and easing patient discomfort. However, biological dressings are only temporary measures; the body eventually rejects them. If the underlying wound hasn't healed, the dressing must be replaced with a graft of the patient's own skin.

Here's a comparison of the four types of biological dressings and their uses.

Type and source	Use and duration	Special considerations
Amnion Made from amnion and chorionic membranes	Used to protect burns and to temporarily cover granulation tissue awaiting a graft. Must be changed every 48 hours.	• Apply only to clean wounds. • Leave open to the air or cover with a dressing.
Biosynthetic Woven from man-made fibers	Used to cover donor sites; to protect clean, superficial burns and excised wounds awaiting grafts; and to cover meshed grafts. Must be reapplied every 3 to 4 days.	• Don't remove to treat the wound (biosynthetic dressings are permeable to antimicrobials).
Heterograft (xenograft) Harvested from animals (usually pigs)	Used to debride untidy wounds, to protect granulation tissue after escharotomy, to protect excisions, to serve as a test graft before skin grafting, and to temporarily cover burns when the patient doesn't have sufficient skin for immediate grafting. Also used to cover meshed grafts, to protect exposed tendons, and to cover burns that are eschar-free and only slightly contaminated. Usually rejected in 7 to 10 days.	• Dress or leave open. • Watch for signs of rejection.
Homograft (allograft) Harvested from cadavers	Used for same purposes as a heterograft. Usually rejected in 7 to 10 days.	• Observe wound for exudate. • Watch for local and systemic signs of rejection.

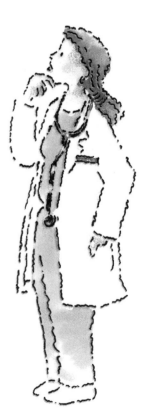

- primary closure would interfere with function
- the wound is on a weight-bearing surface of the body
- a skin tumor is excised and the site needs to be monitored for recurrence.

The three types of skin grafts are:

split-thickness grafts, which consist of the epidermis and a small portion of the dermis

full-thickness grafts, which include the epidermis and all of the dermis

composite grafts, which include the epidermis, dermis, and underlying tissues, such as muscle, cartilage, and bone.

Don't disturb the dressings on your graft and donor sites for any reason. If the dressing needs to be changed, call the doctor.

Secret of success

The success or failure of any skin graft hinges on revascularization. Initially, a skin graft survives by direct contact with the underlying tissue, receiving oxygen and nutrients through existing blood vessels. However, the graft dies unless new blood vessels develop. For split-thickness grafts, revascularization usually takes 3 to 5 days; for full-thickness grafts, up to 2 weeks.

Patient preparation

The graft is taken, or harvested, from an area of healthy tissue on the patient's body. Therefore, it's important to provide meticulous skin care to preserve potential donor sites. Also, because graft survival depends on close contact with underlying tissue, the recipient site — the wound — should be healthy granulation tissue that's free from eschar, debris, and infection.

Aftercare

Afterward, all aspects of care focus on promoting graft survival. Help the patient find comfortable positions for relaxing and sleeping that prevent him from lying on the area of the graft. If feasible, keep the graft elevated and immobilized. When needed, modify your routine to accommodate healing. For example, never use a blood pressure cuff over a graft site. In the case of a burn patient, omit hydrotherapy until the graft heals. Administer analgesics as necessary, but also teach the patient techniques to reduce pain that don't involve medication, such as relaxation techniques.

Always use sterile technique when changing dressings, and work gently to avoid dislodging the graft. Clean the graft site with a warm saline solution and cotton-tipped applicators, leaving the fine-mesh gauze over the graft intact. Aspirate any serous pockets. Change the gauze and apply the prescribed topical agent as needed. Then cover the area with a gauze bandage.

Going home

As the patient prepares to go home, discuss proper care with him. Explain that the dressings on the graft and donor sites shouldn't be disturbed for any reason. If he feels the dressing needs to be changed, he should call the doctor and never attempt it himself. Emphasize that immobilizing the area of the graft is essential for speedy and complete healing. Later, as healing progresses, he can apply cream to the graft site several times per day to keep the skin pliable and help the scar mature.

Sun exposure can affect graft pigmentation. Explain this to your patient and suggest that he limit the amount of time he spends in the sun. Also suggest that he use sun block anytime he plans to be outdoors.

Finally, almost all patients express concern about scarring and appearance. If your patient is worried, explain that if scarring continues to be a problem when the graft completely heals, he can discuss with his doctor plastic surgery options.

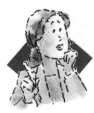

Quick quiz

1. After abdominal surgery, your patient says that he felt something "pop" when he was getting back into bed. You examine his wound and find bowel protruding. You should:
    A.   place the patient in high Fowler's position.
    B.   place the patient in low Fowler's position.
    C.   place the patient flat in bed.
    D.   place the patient on his left side.

Answer: B. Place the patient in low Fowler's position to reduce tension on the wound.

2. What's the first step in caring for a patient with a traumatic wound?
    A.   Get him to the hospital.
    B.   Take a blood pressure measurement.
    C.   Apply pressure bandages.
    D.   Assess his airway, breathing, and circulation.

Answer: D. Your first priority is to assess the patient's airway, breathing, and circulation.

3. When assessing your patient's burns, you note damage to the epidermis and dermis and the presence of black leathery tissue. What type of burn has he suffered?
    A.   First-degree
    B.   Second-degree
    C.   Third-degree
    D.   Fourth-degree

Answer: C. In a third-degree burn, both the epidermis and dermis are damaged. No blisters appear, but eschar and thrombosed vessels may be evident.

4. Which of the following interventions isn't appropriate for a patient with a major burn?
    A.   Remove smoldering clothing.
    B.   Begin I.V. therapy as ordered.
    C.   Cover the burns with a dry, sterile bed sheet.
    D.   Cover the burns with saline-soaked dressings.

Answer: D. Never use cool saline-soaked dressings or towels on a patient with a major burn — body temperature could be drastically reduced resulting in hypothermia.

5. What intervention can best protect the skin around a heavily draining surgical incision from irritation due to wound drainage?
    A.   Pouching
    B.   Packing and gauze dressings
    C.   A hydrocolloid dressing
    D.   An occlusive dressing

Answer: A. Pouching prevents irritation of surrounding tissue when there's copious drainage from an incision.

6. Which of the following statements about skin staples and clips is not a benefit of using them for wound closure?
    A.   They can quickly secure a wound.
    B.   They cause minimal tissue reaction.
    C.   They can be used in areas where good cosmetic results are desirable.
    D.   They can reduce tissue trauma by evenly distributing tension along the suture line.

Answer: C. Because of residual scarring, skin staples and clips aren't used to close a wound if cosmetic results are an issue.

7. Your patient has a surgical wound that has been closed for 8 days. During your wound assessment, you palpate a ridge along the incision line. This ridge may indicate:

    A.   normal healing.

    B.   wound dehiscence.

    C.   wound evisceration.

    D.   wound tunneling.

Answer: A. This ridge, known as the *healing ridge*, is a sign that normal healing is progressing.

Scoring

☆☆☆ If you answered all seven questions correctly, strut your stuff! You've demonstrated acute understanding.

☆☆ If you answered four to six questions correctly, take a bow! Your surgical approach to studying has served you well.

☆ If you answered fewer than four questions correctly, that's okay. We believe you're going to heal quickly.

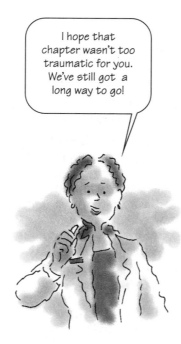

I hope that chapter wasn't too traumatic for you. We've still got a long way to go!

Vascular ulcers

Just the facts

In this chapter, you'll learn:

♦ characteristics of arterial, venous, and lymphatic ulcers

♦ causes for each of these vascular ulcers

♦ assessment criteria for each of these vascular ulcers

♦ treatment options for each of these vascular ulcers, including appropriate dressing types.

A look at vascular ulcers

The vascular system is comprised of arteries, veins, capillaries, and lymphatics. Pressure from the beating heart carries blood away from the heart through the arteries into progressively smaller vessels until they connect with the capillaries. On the other side of the capillaries, small veins receive blood and pass it into progressively larger veins on its return trip to the heart. The lymphatic system is a separate system of vessels that collect waste products and deliver them to the venous system.

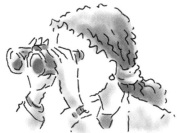

A group of disorders that affect the blood vessels outside the heart, or the lymphatic vessels, are known collectively as peripheral vascular disease (PVD). Vascular ulcers are chronic wounds that stem from PVD in the venous, arterial, and lymphatic systems. Venous and arterial ulcers are most common in the distal lower extremities, whereas lymphatic ulcers occur in the arms or the legs. Let's take a close look at each type.

Venous ulcers

Venous ulcers, which result from venous hypertension, occur on the lower leg. They affect approximately 1% of the population as a whole but are most common in older adults, affecting 3.5% of the population over age 65. Venous ulcers account for 70% to 90% of all leg ulcers.

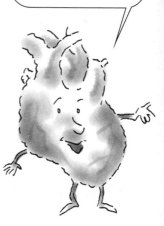

The cardiovascular system is complicated! Nearly 60,000 miles of arteries, arterioles, capillaries, venules, and veins keep blood circulating to and from every functioning cell in the body.

Venous anatomy and function

In the circulatory system, arteries carry blood away from the heart and veins carry blood back to the heart. Capillaries connect these two systems. On the venous side, venules are the small veins that receive blood from the capillaries and deliver it to the larger veins for its return trip to the heart.

Types of veins

In the lower portion of the body, where venous ulcers develop, there are three major types of veins: superficial veins, deep veins, and perforator veins.

Skin deep

Superficial veins lie just beneath the skin and drain into deep veins through perforator veins. Varicose veins are superficial veins that have become stretched and tortuous.

Connectors

Perforator veins connect the superficial veins to the deep veins. Their name is derived from the fact that they perforate the deep fasciae as they connect, like rungs on a ladder, superficial veins to the deep venous system.

Return lanes

Deep veins receive venous blood from the perforator veins and return it to the heart. The major deep veins in the leg include the posterior tibial veins, anterior tibial veins, peroneal veins, and the popliteal veins. Each of these veins parallels a corresponding artery. (See *Major lower limb veins.*)

Vein walls and valves

Compared to arteries of the same size, veins have thinner walls and wider diameters. Vein walls have three distinct layers: an inner, endothelial layer (tunica intima); a middle layer of smooth muscle (tunica media); and an outer, supportive layer (tunica adventitia).

Veins also have a unique system of cup-shaped valves that open toward the heart. The valves function to keep blood flowing in one direction — toward the heart. Deep veins have more of these valves than superficial veins, and veins in the lower leg have

Major lower limb veins

Venous ulcers most commonly occur in the lower extremities. The illustration below shows the major veins in this part of the body.

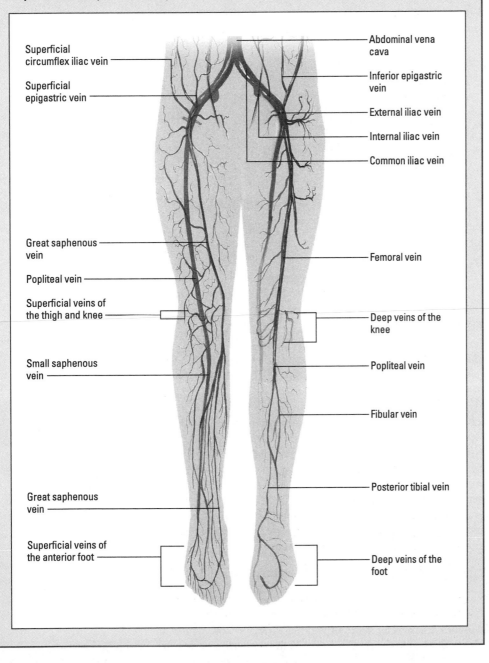

- Superficial circumflex iliac vein
- Superficial epigastric vein
- Great saphenous vein
- Popliteal vein
- Superficial veins of the thigh and knee
- Small saphenous vein
- Great saphenous vein
- Superficial veins of the anterior foot
- Abdominal vena cava
- Inferior epigastric vein
- External iliac vein
- Internal iliac vein
- Common iliac vein
- Femoral vein
- Deep veins of the knee
- Popliteal vein
- Fibular vein
- Posterior tibial vein
- Deep veins of the foot

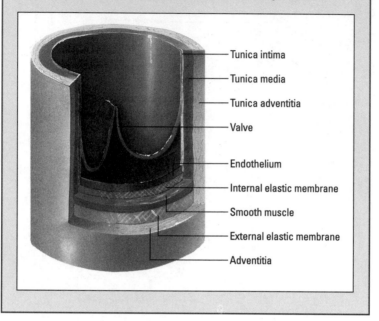

A close look at a vein

This cross section of a vein clearly illustrates the three layers of the vein wall and its unique cup-shaped valves. These valves open toward the heart and, when closed, prevent blood from flowing backward.

- Tunica intima
- Tunica media
- Tunica adventitia
- Valve
- Endothelium
- Internal elastic membrane
- Smooth muscle
- External elastic membrane
- Adventitia

more of these valves than veins in the thigh. In perforator veins, the valves open toward the deep veins. (See *A close look at a vein.*)

Calf muscle pump

Calf muscles have an important role in venous circulation. As calf muscles contract, they squeeze veins in the leg, forcing venous blood toward the heart. When they relax, veins in the leg expand and refill with blood from superficial and perforator veins. This pumping action is important; about 90% of venous blood travels to the heart this way. The other 10% of venous blood empties directly into the vena cava from the great saphenous vein. However, the calf muscles must be active for the calf muscle pump to work. Leg muscle paralysis or prolonged inactivity eliminates the calf muscle pump and inhibits venous blood flow.

Causes

Venous ulcers are the end stage of venous hypertension, which, in turn, results from venous insufficiency. Venous insufficiency simply means that the flow of venous blood from the legs to the heart isn't what it should be. In most cases, incompetent valves are to blame. Valve incompetency may be caused by a thrombus (blood clot) that renders the valve useless or by venous wall distention that separates valve cusps to the point where they no longer meet when the valve closes.

How deep is the problem?

When the flow of venous blood slows, blood pools in the veins of the lower limbs and venous pressure rises. As the disease progresses, blood backs up through the perforator veins into superficial veins, causing varicose veins to develop in the superficial system. In many cases, edema develops as excess interstitial fluid accumulates. Keep in mind, however, that a patient with varicose veins may not have deep vein insufficiency; vascular tests can differentiate between these two problems.

Venous ulcers can occur in patients with superficial or perforator disease as well as those with deep vein disease. In all cases, however, the underlying problem usually is venous hypertension.

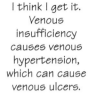

I think I get it. Venous insufficiency causes venous hypertension, which can cause venous ulcers.

Assessment

Proper assessment of venous ulcers includes a thorough history and physical examination.

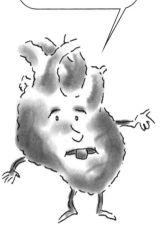

History

Develop a complete history of the patient's experience with venous ulcers. Obtain answers to such questions as:
• When did the patient first notice this ulcer?
• Is this the first time the patient has had an ulcer or is this a recurrence?
• If it's a recurrence, what type of treatment did the patient receive in the past? What type of pain management proved effective?
• Does the patient have a history of varicose veins? Venous thromboses? Arterial disease? Bleeding problems of any type? Leg trauma?
• Does the patient use tobacco?

It may seem like an interrogation, but asking the right questions when taking the patient's history is an important part of assessment.

Physical examination

Record the size of the ulcer (length, width, and depth) and its location. Note any necrosis, drainage, or edema. Record the patient's description of pain associated with the ulcer. Pain may vary from nonexistent to extreme pain.

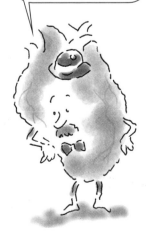

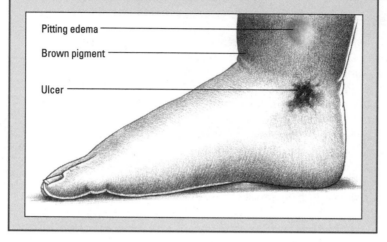

Signs of venous insufficiency

In a patient with venous insufficiency, check for ulcerations around the ankle. Pulses are present but may be difficult to find if edema is present. The foot may become cyanotic when dependent.

Pitting edema

Brown pigment

Ulcer

Venous ulcers may occur anywhere from the ankle to midcalf; however, they're most common on the medial aspect of the ankle above the malleolus and may extend all the way around the leg. Most have an irregular shape. The borders may have dry crusts or be moist and slightly macerated from drainage. The ulcer itself is shallow with a base of beefy red granulation tissue. The surface may be covered by a yellow film or gray necrotic tissue. Black necrotic tissue is rarely present unless an acute injury has occurred. Check for edema and other signs of venous insufficiency. (See *Signs of venous insufficiency*.)

Insufficient data

In venous insufficiency, red blood cells (RBCs), fluid, and fibrin leak into tissues. Note the color of the patient's skin. Hyperpigmentation is common even when ulcers aren't present. This color change is due to a buildup of hemosiderin in the interstitial tissue as the RBCs that have leaked into the tissue break down. The fibrin causes skin and subcutaneous tissue to thicken and become fibrotic — a condition called *lipodermatosclerosis*.

Keep an eye out

Other skin changes characteristic of venous insufficiency include edema, eczema, and atrophie blanche:
• Edema is one of the first signs of venous disease. It may be confined to the foot or the ankle or may involve the entire leg.

• Eczema is common, especially in patients who have recurrent ulcers. Skin over scar tissue and edematous tissue is fragile. Drainage from larger ulcers — or medications themselves — can irritate the skin and aggravate eczema.

• Atrophie blanche may appear as spots of ivory-white plaque in the skin, usually surrounded by hyperpigmentation. Some patients feel discomfort in these areas.

> Watch for skin changes that are characteristic of venous insufficiency, including hyperpigmentation, edema, eczema, and atrophie blanche.

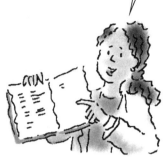

Diagnostic testing

Diagnostic tests for venous ulcers include plethysmography, venous duplex scanning, and venography.

Plethysmography

Plethysmography records changes in the volumes and sizes of extremities by measuring changes in blood volume. There are two types:

• Air plethysmography uses an inflatable pneumatic cuff placed around the limb to obtain volume measurements and standing and walking pressures.

• Photoplethysmography uses infrared light transmitted through the skin to measure venous reflux and filling times. Delayed healing can be predicted by abnormal filling times.

Venous duplex scanning

Venous duplex scanning is used to assess venous patency and reflux by measuring and recording venous pressures along an extremity as its veins are compressed and released. An experienced technician can use venous duplex scanning to identify thrombosis within a vein and determine whether it's acute or chronic as well as assess venous reflux and the status of valve function. The accuracy of the results depends entirely on the technician's skill.

Venography

Venography is the radiographic examination of a vein injected with a contrast medium. For a long time, this was the only test available to evaluate venous thrombosis. However, with the advent of newer noninvasive tests, venography is rarely used anymore.

Treatment

Effective treatment of a venous ulcer involves caring for the wound and managing the underlying venous disease. Controlling edema is the most important goal in managing chronic venous insufficiency. Methods to accomplish this include elevation of the affected limb, compression therapy and, sometimes, medication or surgery. Wound care involves selecting the best dressing for a venous ulcer.

Get a leg up! The most effective method of reducing edema in a patient with venous ulcers is to raise the affected extremity higher than the heart.

Elevation of the limb

The most effective method of reducing edema is to elevate the leg and allow gravity to drain fluid from the limb. This is best accomplished with the patient in bed with his legs elevated above the level of his heart. However, a patient with a cardiac or pulmonary condition may find this position intolerable. In this case, any elevation that the patient can tolerate is beneficial.

Compression therapy

Compression bandages are useful when a patient can't elevate the affected limb. They're also helpful for times when a patient is on his feet. Finding the right bandage isn't hard; various rigid and flexible models are available. However, before a compression bandage is added to the treatment regimen, assess ankle brachial index (ABI) to ensure the adequacy of arterial supply. (For more information, see the section on assessing ABI later in this chapter.)

Unna's boot

Unna's boot, a commercially prepared, inelastic, medicated gauze compression bandage, is one of the oldest treatments for venous ulcers. It's one of the most widely used compression bandages because it's inexpensive and effective. This dressing is especially useful for patients who pick at sores, because it renders the ulcer inaccessible. The dressing should be changed weekly, or more frequently if needed.

Unna's boot consists of a gauze roll that's impregnated with zinc oxide, calamine, and glycerin and placed over the skin from below the toes to just below the knee. Any concavity over the ulcer is filled with additional dressing. This dressing is covered with cotton dressings to pad the wound and to absorb drainage. An elastic bandage is wrapped around the outside to provide compression. As the dressing dries, it becomes semirigid. (See *How to wrap Unna's boot.*)

Featuring...rigidity

Although Unna's boot provides compression, protection, and a moist environment for healing, its most significant feature is its

Dress for success

How to wrap Unna's boot

To wrap an Unna's boot, follow these steps:
• Clean the patient's skin thoroughly and then flex his knee.
• With the foot positioned at a right angle to the leg, wrap the medicated gauze bandage firmly—not tightly—around the patient's foot. Make sure the dressing covers the heel.
• Continue wrapping upward, overlapping the layers by 50% with each turn. Make sure the dressing circles the leg at an angle to avoid compromising the circulation. Smooth the boot with your free hand as you go, as shown top right.
• Stop wrapping about 1″ (2.5 cm) below the knee, as shown bottom right. If constriction develops as the dressing hardens, make a 2″ (5.1 cm) slit in the boot just below the knee.
• If drainage is excessive, wrap a roller gauze dressing over the boot.
• Finally, wrap the boot with an elastic bandage in a figure-eight pattern.

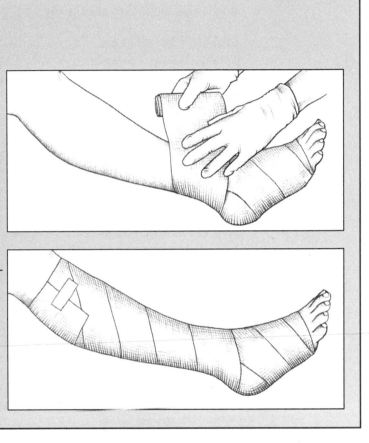

rigidity. Calf muscle contractions are key to the effectiveness of Unna's boot. As the patient walks, the rigid dressing restricts outward movement of the calf muscle, directing more of the contraction force inward and improving the function of the calf muscle pump and, in turn, venous circulation. Therefore, Unna's boot is much less effective for a sedentary or bedridden patient. If the patient finds the firmness against the ulcer uncomfortable, place a hydrocolloid or foam dressing over the ulcer before applying Unna's boot.

Compression stockings

Compression stockings are essential for long-term management of lower extremity venous disease. They're available in four classes of pressure, as measured at the ankle. Each package of stockings has a list of indications on the label; however, most health care professionals rely on their own experience when choosing a class for a specific patient with a specific problem. Be aware that a patient with arthritis, back problems, or obesity may have problems donning compression stockings.

CircAid Thera-Boot

If Unna's boot or compression stockings aren't viable options, a CircAid Thera-Boot may be the answer. This dressing provides approximately 30 to 40 mm Hg of compression and is easier to put on than compression stockings, as long as the patient can bend down to reach his legs. The CircAid Thera-Boot is made of a nonelastic semirigid material and has easy-to-use straps that secure the dressing in place. This dressing is washable and reusable and can be removed at night and then put back on in the morning.

Layered compression bandages

Layered compression bandages with three or four layers are relatively new additions to the list of dressing options. In these bandages, the first layer is cotton wool, which protects the skin and absorbs moisture. This layer can be pulled apart and repositioned to fill concavities and create a more uniform fit. In some versions, a support bandage is the next layer. This layer provides a smooth surface for the compression layers above. Above this is a light compression bandage that provides about 17 mm Hg of pressure. The final layer is a compression bandage that provides 23 mm Hg of pressure.

Elastic bandages

Elastic bandages are inexpensive wraps that may be used for compression. They may be short- or long-stretch.

The short...

A short-stretch bandage has limited elastic stretch, typically less than 90% of its length. When stretched to its limit, a short-stretch bandage becomes semirigid, providing compression while the patient is active. When the patient rests, the dressing provides less compression, protecting the skin from unnecessary pressure. This type of bandage is characterized as providing high working pressure and low resting pressure.

...and long of it

A long-stretch bandage stretches to more than 140% of its length. Long-stretch bandages provide low working pressure and high resting pressure. A long-stretch bandage exerts a specific amount of pressure all the time, whether the patient is active or resting and may provide more pressure than is desirable during periods of rest.

> Sometimes layers are a must. Layered compression bandages protect the skin, absorb moisture, and provide compression.

Graduated compression support hosiery

As their name suggests, graduated compression support stockings provide a pressure gradient that's greatest at the ankle and lowest at the top of the stocking. This compression is consistent with the hydrostatic pressure in leg veins, which is greatest at the ankle and then diminishes up the leg. These stockings exert 100% of their pressure at the ankle, 70% at the calf, and 40% at the thigh level, producing a pressure gradient that helps reduce venous reflux. Knee-high length stockings are all that's necessary to prevent venous ulcers.

Compression pumps may be used in conjunction with support hosiery. These devices are available with sleeves that intermittently inflate. They may have a single chamber or separate bladders that inflate sequentially.

Medication

Medications are rarely prescribed to treat venous ulcers. Antibiotics may be ordered to treat infection. In most instances, they're given systemically because topical antibiotics aren't effective in treating wound infections; in fact, they may interfere with healing. Also, if the patient is a candidate for skin grafting, topical antibiotics may be used to kill surface bacteria before the procedure.

Diuretics shouldn't be prescribed to treat edema in cases of venous insufficiency because edema is typically treated in these cases with compression and limb elevation. If the patient has concomitant heart failure, diuretics may be prescribed to treat that condition. Because diuretics can cause volume depletion and serious metabolic disorders, monitor the patient closely.

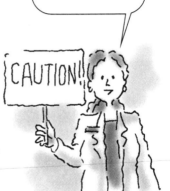

If diuretics are prescribed to treat a patient with concomitant heart failure, monitor the patient carefully for volume depletion and metabolic disorders.

Surgery

Venous ulcers are a chronic disorder. As such, they're slow to heal and recur frequently. Consequently, surgery is rarely a viable treatment. Large surface defects may require repair by skin grafting, but this is a temporary solution. The underlying problem of venous hypertension remains and, in time, edema beneath the scar tissue breaks down the scar and creates another ulcer.

Replacement parts

Valve transplant, which involves replacing a section of vein containing a defective valve with a section of vein containing a healthy valve, is performed selectively and almost never for a patient with venous ulcers. This is because by the time an ulcer forms venous disease is so pervasive that replacing a single valve won't help.

Success of SEPS

Another surgical procedure called subfascial endoscopic perforator surgery (SEPS) may be performed more often. In SEPS, which is based on the theory that incompetent perforator veins cause ulcers at the ankles, faulty perforator veins are located and ligated, redirecting blood flow to healthy veins and improving ulcer healing.

Wound care

Choosing the proper dressing is an important part of wound care because it affects wound healing. Occlusive dressings are typically selected for venous ulcers because they promote growth of granulation tissue and reepithelialization. If an ulcer contains necrotic debris, a moist gauze dressing or hydrocolloid dressing can be used to provide autolytic debridement. It's appropriate to select a dressing that promotes moist wound healing even though venous ulcers typically produce copious amounts of drainage. Hydrocolloid dressings, transparent films, and some foam dressings retain moisture in the wound while absorbing light to moderate drainage. More absorbent dressings can be used for venous ulcers with moderate to heavy drainage.

And introducing...

Newer therapies can also aid in healing chronic venous ulcers. Preliminary studies show that growth factors can be used to improve the healing rate in venous ulcers. In addition, a bioengineered skin equivalent called Apligraf can be used on venous ulcers that fail to heal within 4 weeks of treatment. (For more information on adjunctive therapies, see chapter 9, Therapeutic modalities.)

Arterial ulcers

Arterial ulcers, which are also called ischemic ulcers, are the result of tissue ischemia due to arterial insufficiency. They can occur at the distal (farthest) end of any arterial branch, and they account for 5% to 20% of all leg ulcers.

Arterial anatomy and function

Like vein walls, artery walls have three layers:

The tunica intima, the innermost layer, is a single layer of endothelial cells on a layer of connective tissue.

A close look at an artery

This cross section of an artery illustrates the layers that comprise the arterial wall.

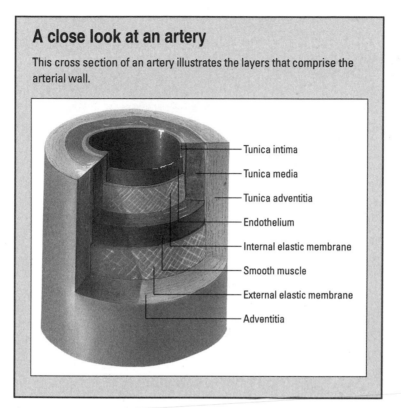

- Tunica intima
- Tunica media
- Tunica adventitia
- Endothelium
- Internal elastic membrane
- Smooth muscle
- External elastic membrane
- Adventitia

The tunica media, the middle layer, is a thick layer of smooth-muscle cells, collagen, and elastic fibers.

The tunica adventitia, the strong outer layer, is comprised of connective tissue, collagen, and elastic fibers. (See *A close look at an artery*.)

With every beat of my heart

Arteries carry blood leaving the heart to every functioning cell in the body. Their strong, muscular walls allow arteries to expand and relax with each heartbeat, smoothing the powerful pulse to an almost constant pressure by the time blood reaches the capillaries. The lower portion of the body receives its arterial flow through the abdominal aorta and the major arteries that branch from it. (See *Major lower limb arteries*, page 110.)

Causes

Arterial insufficiency occurs when arterial blood flow is interrupted by an obstruction or by narrowing of an artery (arterial steno-

Major lower limb arteries

This illustration identifies the major arteries in the lower portion of the body.

Aorta

Superficial circumflex iliac artery

Medial femoral circumflex artery

Lateral femoral circumflex artery

Deep femoral artery

Perforating branch

Medial superior genicular artery

Medial inferior genicular artery

Deep plantar arterial arch

Dorsal metatarsal arteries

Dorsal digital arteries

Gonadal artery

Common iliac artery

Internal iliac artery

External iliac artery

Femoral artery

Descending genicular artery

Lateral superior genicular artery

Popliteal artery

Lateral inferior genicular artery

Anterior tibial artery

Peroneal artery

Posterior tibial artery

Dorsalis pedis artery

Lateral tarsal artery

Lateral plantar artery

Arcuate artery

sis). Occlusion can occur in any artery—from the aorta to a capillary—and can result from trauma or chronic ailment. In time, arterial insufficiency leads to arterial ulcers.

The origins of occlusion

The most common cause of occlusion is atherosclerosis. Those patients at highest risk for atherosclerosis include males, cigarette smokers, and individuals with diabetes mellitus, hyperlipidemia, or hypertension. Advanced age places patients at even greater risk because, as aging occurs, the tunica intima thickens and loses elasticity. Thickening of the intima is one cause of arterial stenosis.

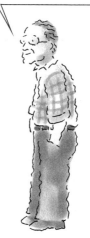

Thickening of the tunica intima, which occurs normally with aging, is one cause of arterial stenosis. This puts me at greater risk for arterial insufficiency.

Warning signs

In many cases, no signs of arterial insufficiency are apparent until the affected individual suffers an injury. As the demand for additional blood flow to the site of the injury outpaces an occluded artery's ability to deliver it, ischemia occurs. Ischemia is a reduction in the flow of blood to any organ or body part. The primary symptom of ischemia is pain, and this pain can be severe. This pain may progress from claudication to rest pain.

Claudication

Claudication has been described as "angina of the leg muscles" because the cause of both is an insufficient supply of oxygen. In heart muscle, this deficiency causes the pain of angina. In leg muscles, the same deficiency causes the pain of claudication.

Claudication, which can occur in any muscle distal to a narrowed artery, is brought on by exercise and is relieved by rest. Typically, patients report claudication pain in the calf, thigh, or buttocks. It's measured by how many city blocks (or equivalent distance) the patient can walk before needing to stop to relieve the pain. Factors that tend to shorten the distance traveled before pain occurs include obesity, smoking, and progressive atherosclerotic disease.

Claudication occurs at a specific distance and is reproducible. Unlike angina, patients experiencing claudication don't have to sit or adopt a particular position to relieve the discomfort; merely stopping reduces the oxygen demand and relieves the pain. As arterial insufficiency progresses, the distance shortens until, ultimately, the patient feels pain even when resting.

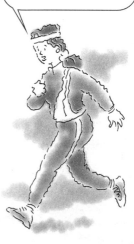

Claudication pain in the calf, thigh, or buttocks that's brought on by exercise and is relieved by rest may be the first sign of arterial insufficiency.

Rest pain

Rest pain commonly occurs in the foot and can occur when the patient is asleep. Getting up and walking may provide some relief; however, walking isn't the key — lowering the extremity is. Gravity helps blood flow into the foot and calf, reducing the oxygen deficit and relieving discomfort. By the time rest pain occurs, tissues in the foot are severely ischemic, whether or not an ulcer is present. Unless arterial flow is restored, the patient may face amputation.

> Rest pain in the foot is more likely to be reduced by lowering the foot than by walking. Gravity helps blood flow into the foot, reducing the oxygen deficit and relieving discomfort.

Assessment

Assessment of arterial ulcers requires a thorough patient history and physical examination.

History

A patient history reveals whether the patient's wound is an arterial ulcer caused by arterial insufficiency.

What a pain!

Ask the patient whether he's experienced any pain. If he describes intermittent claudication, ask him to estimate how far he can walk before pain sets in. If the patient says he has pain while resting, ask him when he first noticed it and what measures he takes to relieve the pain. If the pain is in the foot, ask if getting up or hanging that foot over the edge of the bed helps. Ask the patient what position is most comfortable. Many patients spend their nights sleeping in a chair because the arterial pressure in the leg is too low to perfuse tissues while the leg is extended.

Smoke signals

Ask about smoking as well. If the patient smokes, determine how long he's been a smoker and how much he smokes.

Physical examination

Start the examination by inspecting the common sites of arterial ulcers: the tips of toes, the corners of nail beds on the toes, over bony prominences, and between toes. The edges of arterial ulcers are well demarcated. Because there's little blood flow to the tissue, the base of the ulcer is pale and dry, and no granulation tissue is present. There may be an area of wet necrosis or a dry scab.

Signs of arterial insufficiency

Arterial ulcers most commonly occur in the area around the toes. In a patient with arterial insufficiency, the foot usually turns deep red when dependent and the nails may be thick and ridged. In addition, pulses may be faint or absent; the skin is cool, pale, and shiny; and the patient may report pain in his legs and feet.

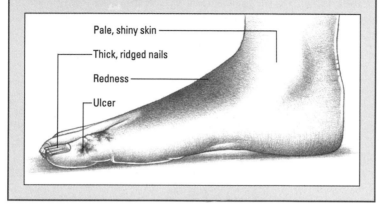

Pale, shiny skin

Thick, ridged nails

Redness

Ulcer

The skin surrounding the ulcer feels cooler than normal on palpation. (See *Signs of arterial insufficiency*.)

Next, elevate the foot with the ulcer to a 30-degree angle; the skin color in an ischemic foot pales. Then ask the patient to place his foot in a dependent position. Ischemic skin becomes deep red as the tissue refills with blood. This dramatic color change is called *dependent rubor*—a sign of severe tissue ischemia. The nails may be thin and pale yellow, or they may have thickened due to an existing fungal infection in the nail beds. A Doppler signal may be heard over small arteries, but this doesn't signify blood flow that's sufficient enough to heal the ulcer.

Focus pocus

Perform a focused examination of the arterial system. Palpate the abdominal aorta for the presence of an aortic aneurysm. (In an obese patient, this won't be palpable.) An embolus can occlude an artery and cause ischemia, and an aortic aneurysm may be the source of the embolus. "Blue toe syndrome," a painful, ischemic toe, is caused by embolic debris in the arteries that supply the toe.

Palpate the femoral, popliteal, posterior tibial, and dorsalis pedis pulses in each leg and compare your findings. (See *Assessing lower extremity pulses*, page 114.) Keep in mind that an absent dorsalis pedis pulse may not be an abnormal finding. Under normal conditions, some patients don't have a palpable dorsalis pedis pulse. Pulses can be palpated when the pressure is about

Assessing lower extremity pulses

The following illustrations show where to position your fingers when palpating for pulses of the lower extremities. Use your index and middle fingers to apply pressure.

Femoral pulse

Press relatively hard at a point inferior to the inguinal ligament. For an obese patient, palpate in the crease of the groin, halfway between the pubic bone and the hip bone.

Popliteal pulse

Press firmly in the popliteal fossa at the back of the knee.

Posterior tibial pulse

Apply pressure behind and slightly below the medial malleolus.

Dorsalis pedis pulse

Place your fingers on the medial dorsum of the foot while the patient points his toes down. The pulse is difficult to palpate here and may seem to be absent in healthy patients.

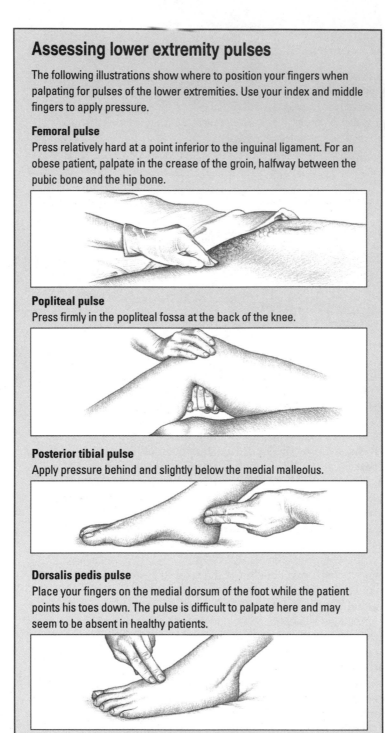

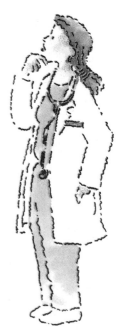

80 mm Hg. If there's no palpable pulse, the pressure is probably less than 80 mm Hg. Pulses aren't palpable in a foot with an arterial ulcer.

Compare the color of both legs and palpate each for temperature. A difference in temperature of 10 degrees or more can be noted by palpation. While the patient lies down, elevate both of his feet about 12″ (30.5 cm), or to a 30-degree angle. Watch for a color change. Compress the great toe bilaterally and compare the capillary refill of each side. Normal tissue should refill in less than 3 seconds.

> Taking blood pressure measurements in the arms and legs is a good way to assess the adequacy of arterial blood flow to the legs.

Diagnostic tests

Diagnostic tests commonly used to assess arterial flow to the extremities include segmental pressure recordings, Doppler ultrasonography, ABI, transcutaneous oxygen measurement, and arteriography.

Segmental pressure recordings

Blood pressure is the first test performed to assess the adequacy of arterial blood flow to the legs. Normally, blood pressure readings taken in the arm and the leg should be the same when the patient is lying down. A lower reading in the legs indicates an arterial blockage that may be caused by such problems as a thrombus, cholesterol, or pressure on the outside of the artery.

Blood pressure is measured in both arms while the patient is lying down. Then blood pressure is measured at several points along each leg. Each reading is accompanied by a waveform tracing of the pulse at the time. The entire procedure takes only 20 to 30 minutes. In some cases, the procedure is repeated after a short period of controlled exercise. In arterial insufficiency, arterial blood flow during exercise fails to keep up with the demand of the muscles. Changes in the waveforms and Doppler signals should occur at the same time the patient reports symptoms of claudication.

Doppler ultrasonography

In Doppler ultrasonography, sound waves are used to assess blood flow. This test may be used alone or in conjunction with other diagnostic tests to assess arterial blood flow. During the procedure, a handheld transducer directs high-frequency

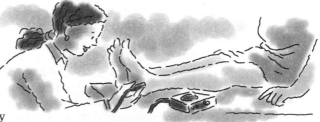

Now I get it!

How the Doppler probe works

The Doppler ultrasound probe directs high-frequency sound waves through layers of tissue. When the sound waves strike red blood cells (RBCs) moving in the bloodstream, the frequency of the sound waves changes in proportion to the velocity of the RBCs. A recording of these waves facilitates detection of arterial and venous obstruction.

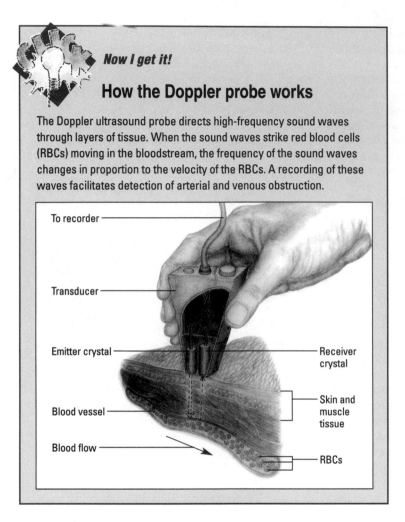

sound waves into the artery being tested. Sound waves that strike moving RBCs change frequency—a Doppler shift—in relation to the velocity of the RBCs. The doctor then reviews the graphic record of these waveforms to determine whether an obstruction exists. (See *How the Doppler probe works*.)

Ankle-brachial index

ABI is a value derived from blood pressure measurements that, taken as a whole, illustrate the progress of arterial disease—or degree of improvement—in the affected limb. Each value in the index is a ratio of a blood pressure measurement in the affected limb to the systolic blood pressure in the brachial arteries. Improvement, or lack thereof, becomes clear when the most recent value is compared to prior values.

The index can also be used to assess treatment methods. Comparing a reading taken before surgery, such as bypass surgery or angioplasty, to a reading taken afterward can indicate the procedure's effectiveness.

How it works

When measuring ABI, a Doppler ultrasound and a blood pressure cuff are employed. The steps of the procedure are as follows:
• First, the patient is placed in a horizontal position so the brachial artery and the dorsalis pedis and posterior tibial arteries are at the same level.
• Next, brachial blood pressure measurements are taken on both sides. If they differ, the higher of the two systolic pressures is used to calculate the ABI.
• Then the blood pressure cuff is wrapped around the ankle just above the malleoli. The dorsalis pedis or posterior tibial artery is identified, and the Doppler transducer is held over the artery at a 45-degree angle.
• The blood pressure cuff is inflated until the Doppler signal is no longer heard; then the cuff is slowly deflated. When the Doppler signal returns, the pressure is recorded. This is the ankle systolic pressure.
• ABI is calculated by dividing the ankle pressure by the higher of the two brachial systolic pressures. (See *Interpreting ABI results*.)

> ### Interpreting ABI results
>
> This chart will help you interpret ankle-brachial index (ABI) calculations. Keep in mind that ABI results aren't reliable for patients with diabetes.
>
> | ABI | Interpretation |
> | --- | --- |
> | > 0.9 | Normal |
> | 0.5 to 0.9 | Claudication |
> | < 0.5 | Resting ischemic pain |
> | < 0.2 | Gangrene |

Transcutaneous oxygen measurement

Some vascular laboratories perform transcutaneous oxygen measurement to assess the perfusion of the microvasculature.

In this test, an electrode is attached to the patient's skin using double-sided tape. Room temperature is kept constant to ensure an accurate reading. Then the patient is monitored for approximately 20 minutes as the measurement is taken.

A transcutaneous oxygen of approximately 40 mm Hg is generally regarded as the cutoff value associated with inability to heal. However, the accuracy and, in turn, the dependability of this test varies.

Arteriogram

Arteriography is an invasive procedure that's only performed if the patient agrees to undergo a corrective procedure for any problem discovered. It's obtained by inserting a catheter into the arterial system, injecting a radiopaque contrast medium (a contrast medium that X-rays can't pass through), and

> Using a radiopaque contrast medium and X-rays, arteriography produces an image of the arteries that can be used to detect defects.

taking an X-ray as the contrast medium is injected. The resulting image shows the lumen of the artery and any defect present.

The procedure carries drawbacks and some significant risks. For example, several medications can't be taken for a time before the procedure. Also, some patients may be allergic to the contrast medium. Possible complications include injury to the artery that requires emergency surgery and hematoma that requires drainage.

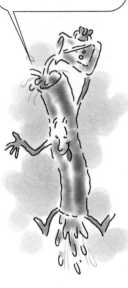

The first goal of treatment of arterial ulcers is to reestablish arterial flow. This can be achieved through bypass surgery or angioplasty and stents.

Treatment

The first goal in treatment of an arterial ulcer is reestablishing arterial flow. Without oxygenated blood, the ulcer won't heal. Options for revascularization include arterial bypass surgery or angioplasty and stents. In addition, the ulcer must receive appropriate wound care. In general, medications aren't effective when arterial insufficiency has advanced to the point that ulcers are present.

Arterial bypass

Arterial bypass is the most common method of restoring arterial flow. The type and extent of bypass surgery depends on the disease's stage and location and the patient's general health. The graft may be autogenous (a vessel taken from the patient) or a synthetic material, typically Dacron or polytetrafluorene.

Angioplasty and stents

Less-invasive interventions, such as angioplasty, are becoming more commonly used than surgery for treatment of arterial stenosis. During angioplasty, a catheter with a balloon is inserted into the patient's artery. Using fluoroscopy, the surgeon carefully maneuvers the catheter to the portion of the artery narrowed by plaque and then expands the balloon. The expanding balloon crushes the plaque against the wall of the artery, increasing the lumen diameter.

Stents are small metal structures that can be inserted into an artery after angioplasty to hold the artery open. They were developed to extend the amount of time the artery remains open after angioplasty and, with luck, reduce the need for surgery. Stent placement is still relatively new, and the success rate of this procedure over time has yet to be determined. However, stents may be an alternative for a patient who's considered too high risk for surgery.

(Text continues on page 119.)

Vascular ulcers

Vascular ulcers typically result from some form of peripheral vascular disease, which can affect the arterial, venous, and lymphatic systems.

Venous ulcers

Venous ulcers result from venous hypertension. These ulcers, the most frequently occurring lower leg ulcers, are typically found around the ankle, as shown in the photo below.

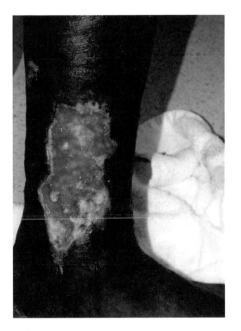

Lymphatic ulcers

Lymphatic ulcers result from lymphedema, in which the capillaries are compressed by thickened tissue, which occludes blood flow to the skin. Lymphatic ulcers are extremely difficult to treat because of this reduced blood flow. The photo below shows a patient with lymphedema of the leg and a large lymphatic ulcer.

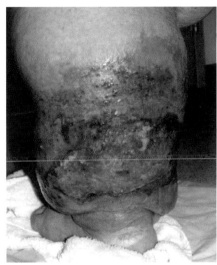

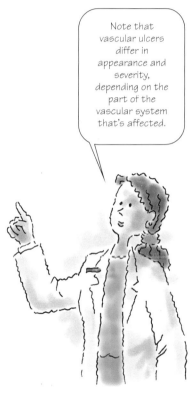

Note that vascular ulcers differ in appearance and severity, depending on the part of the vascular system that's affected.

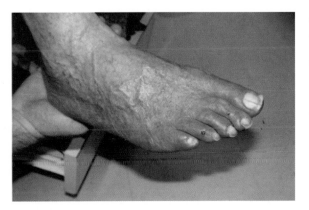

Arterial ulcers

Arterial ulcers result from insufficient blood flow to tissue due to arterial insufficiency. They're commonly found at the distal ends of arterial branches, especially at the tips of the toes, the corners of nail beds, or over bony prominences, as shown in the photo at left.

Staging pressure ulcers

You can use pressure ulcer characteristics gained from your assessment to stage the pressure ulcer, as described here. Staging reflects the anatomic depth of exposed tissue. Keep in mind that if the wound contains necrotic tissue, you won't be able to determine the stage until you can see the wound base.

Welcome hither, and learn thee of pressure ulcer stages. As Shakespeare knew, all the world's a stage...

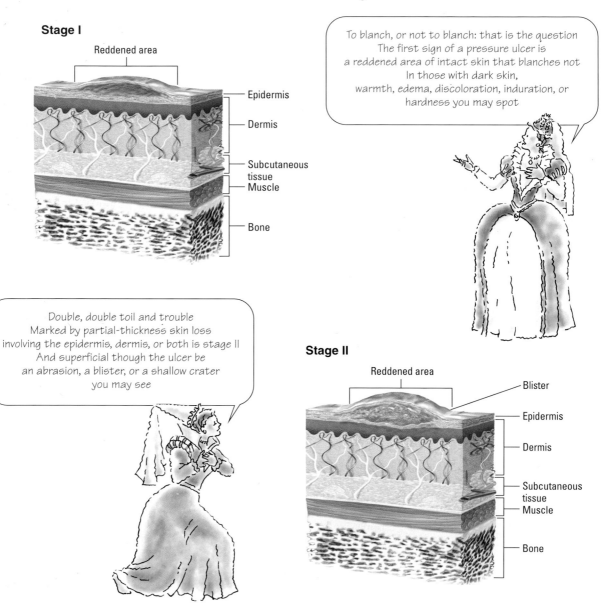

Stage I

Reddened area

Epidermis

Dermis

Subcutaneous tissue

Muscle

Bone

*To blanch, or not to blanch: that is the question
The first sign of a pressure ulcer is
a reddened area of intact skin that blanches not
In those with dark skin,
warmth, edema, discoloration, induration, or
hardness you may spot*

*Double, double toil and trouble
Marked by partial-thickness skin loss
involving the epidermis, dermis, or both is stage II
And superficial though the ulcer be
an abrasion, a blister, or a shallow crater
you may see*

Stage II

Reddened area

Blister

Epidermis

Dermis

Subcutaneous tissue

Muscle

Bone

Stage III

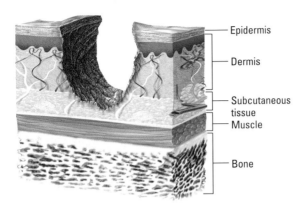

- Epidermis
- Dermis
- Subcutaneous tissue
- Muscle
- Bone

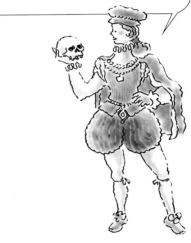

Now is the winter of our discontent
In stage III, the ulcer is a full-thickness wound
that appears like a deep crater when inspected
Underlying fasciae it may extend to
and thou might find undermining of the tissue
that's connected

That it should come to this!
As through the skin the ulcer extends,
damage to muscle, bone, and supporting structures
accompany necrosis of tissues
Alas, undermining and sinus tracts
may also be issues

Stage IV

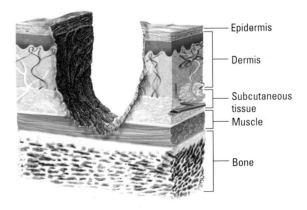

- Epidermis
- Dermis
- Subcutaneous tissue
- Muscle
- Bone

Parting is such sweet sorrow, that I shall say, "Go forth and provide good wound care for all morrows!"

Diabetic foot ulcers

Because of the neurologic and vascular complications associated with diabetes, patients with this disorder are prone to foot ulcers. As with other pressure ulcers, diabetic foot ulcers typically develop over bony prominences when pressure is unrelieved.

This photo shows a patient with diabetes who has a pressure wound to the right lateral malleoli. Note the characteristic tissue changes associated with arterial insufficiency: thin, shiny skin; pale coloring; and muscular atrophy in the lower extremity.

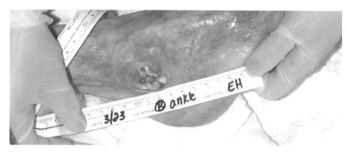

This photo shows a patient with type II diabetes who has developed a pressure ulcer from impaired protective sensation and poor mobility.

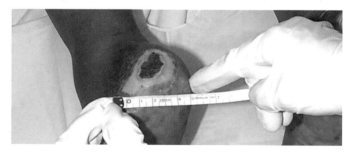

This photo shows a patient who has a diabetic foot ulcer on the plantar surface of the fifth metatarsal head. The circular shape of the wound is consistent with a wound created by pressure over a bony prominence.

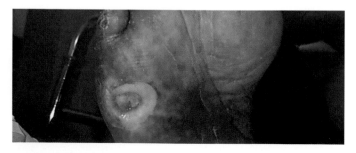

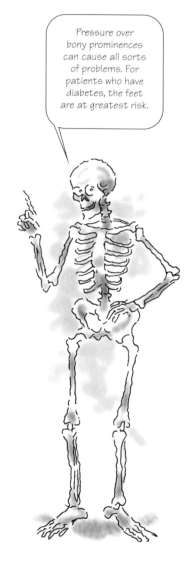

> Pressure over bony prominences can cause all sorts of problems. For patients who have diabetes, the feet are at greatest risk.

Wound care

Keep arterial ulcers dry and protected from pressure. For toe ulcers, place small alcohol pads between the toes and change them daily. As the alcohol dries, it promotes a dry ulcer bed. Never soak arterial ulcers. Ischemic tissue macerates in water, increasing the extent of tissue loss, and promoting bacterial proliferation.

Foot fetish

Make sure the patient's foot is protected at all times. Consider using a large bulky dressing or protective footgear—there are many types to choose from. Keep in mind that ischemic tissue can easily develop additional ulcers with little irritation or pressure. Even pressure from the foot resting on the bed or an ill-fitting protective boot can initiate new ulcers. If your patient opts for foot protection, check the device carefully for possible pressure points.

If the ulcer area contains necrotic tissue or develops dry gangrene, continue to apply a dry dressing. Reassure the patient that a necrotic digit won't cause further harm. However, these areas have no sensation and must be protected from injury. If loss of a toe seems imminent, explain this to the patient and let him talk about his feelings. Having a necrotic toe fall off is a shocking and frightening event for most patients, but it's even more devastating when the patient isn't prepared for it.

Toe the line

Carefully monitor the line of demarcation between dead and viable tissues. This area is typically painful and is easily infected. Treat infected ischemic tissue with I.V. antibiotics.

If revascularization succeeds, it's time to change the type of dressing. At this point, you can treat the wound according to the axiom, "keep moist tissues moist and dry tissues dry." Use any dressing that keeps the wound bed moist and the surrounding tissue dry. Consider using a hydrocolloid or hydrogel dressing. Use a moist dressing in the wound bed and cover this with a dry dressing for protection. When securing the dressing, remember to tape from one area of the dressing to another—not to the patient's skin.

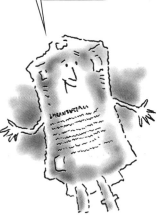

Ischemic tissue that becomes infected may need to be treated with I.V. antibiotics.

Lymphatic ulcers

Lymphatic ulcers, which result from injury in the presence of lymphedema, occur most commonly on the arms and legs. Lymphedema leaves the skin vulnerable to infection and creates skin folds that trap moisture. These conditions cause ulcerations that become difficult to treat.

Lymphatic anatomy and function

The lymphatic system is a component of the peripheral vascular system. Lymph is a protein rich fluid similar to plasma. As lymph circulates through lymphatic vessels, it collects wastes, including bacteria, and transports them to lymph nodes. The nodes filter wastes out of the lymph and add lymphocytes to the fluid. Lymph moves slowly through the lymphatic system, driven by muscle contraction and filtration.

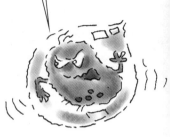

How do you like that?! The lymphatic system circulates lymph through vessels to the lymph nodes, where wastes, including bacteria like me, are filtered.

Causes

Lymphedema is swelling that results when an obstruction prevents the normal flow of lymph into venous circulation. Injury to the swollen tissue may cause an ulcer that's slow to heal.

Lymphedema may be congenital or acquired. Acquired lymphedema can be caused by surgery that severs or removes lymph nodes—radical mastectomy, for example—or it may result from compression of a vessel or node due to obesity or unrelated chronic swelling. For instance, patients with chronic venous hypertension and insufficiency may eventually develop lymphedema if venous edema is poorly managed.

Patients with lymphedema are prone to skin and soft tissue infections and may require long-term treatment with antibiotics. Prophylactic treatment with antibiotics isn't uncommon, because lymphedema causes progressive destruction of lymphatic vessels and nodes which, in turn, slowly increases the patient's risk of infection. Recurrent cellulitis (tissue inflammation) is common.

Hard to handle

In the legs, lymphedema causes a steady seepage of fluids into interstitial tissue. In time, skin and underlying tissues become firm and fibrotic. Thickened tissue presses on the capillaries and occludes blood flow to the skin. The resulting poor circulation makes the leg ulcers that occur with lymphedema extremely difficult to treat.

Leg ulcers on lymphedematous tissue are usually the result of traumatic injury or pressure. However, in extreme cases of lymphedema, the folds of tissue develop deep fissures that trap moisture, causing tissue maceration and the start of a new ulcer.

Assessment

Lymphatic ulcers are most common in the ankle area but may develop at any trauma site. Ulcers are shallow and may be oozing, moist, or blistered. The surrounding skin is usually firm, fibrotic, and thickened by edema. Cellulitis may be present as well. A diagnosis of lymphedema is based on the clinical appearance of the skin.

Treatment

Treatment of lymphatic ulcers has two goals:

☞ to reduce edema (and maintain the reduction)

☞ to prevent complications such as infection.

Leg elevation is an important part of therapy for patients with lymphedema. However, in cases of long-standing edema, elevation may be ineffective.

Support hose and pumps

A compression pump is another effective method of reducing edema; however, pump use becomes a lifelong part of managing edema. The pump reduces the volume of fluid in a lymphedematous limb. The pressure should be set low, in the range of 30 to 50 mm Hg. After each compression session, patients must put on compression bandages or another compression garment. Without these, progress gained from the pumping is lost as soon as the patient stands or sits upright.

Comprehensive decongestive therapy is a form of massage that has proven effective for some patients. After each session, the affected limb is wrapped with a short-stretch bandage.

Wound care

Wound care for lymphatic leg ulcers is similar to care for venous ulcers. The primary difference is that the risk of infection is much higher for patients with lymphedema. In lymphedema, choose dressings that can manage large fluid loads while protecting surrounding skin, such as foams or other absorbent dressings.

Vascular ulcer care wrap-up

Keep the following tips in mind as you care for a patient with any form of vascular ulcer:

• The ulcer is only the tip of the iceberg. Care must also address the underlying disorder or the ulcer won't heal. For instance, with venous ulcers, the underlying venous hypertension must be treated. With arterial ulcers, arterial blood flow must be restored.

• Vascular disease is pervasive, so look for problems in other areas of the body.

Dress for success

Dressings for vascular ulcers

Choosing the best type of dressing for your patient's vascular ulcer depends not only on the ulcer type but also on its condition. The chart below lists indications and contraindications for each dressing according to ulcer type.

To use the chart, find the type of ulcer you're trying to dress and then look down the column for indications and contraindications for each dressing type. For example, the chart indicates that an alginate dressing can be used to manage copious drainage in a venous ulcer but isn't indicated for arterial ulcers.

Dressing	Indications and contraindications		
	Venous ulcers	*Arterial ulcers*	*Lymphatic ulcers*
Alginates	• Use to manage copious drainage.	• Not indicated	• Not indicated
Foam	• Use to protect the ulcer. • Use for absorption underneath a compression dressing.	• Use to protect the ulcer. • Use with dry gangrene. • Use for a moist, revascularized ulcer.	• Use to protect the ulcer. • Use to absorb drainage.
Gauze	• Use for absorption.	• Use for protection and to allow dry gangrene to maintain its dryness.	• Use for absorption or padding. (Don't allow to dry out on the ulcer.)
Hydrocolloids	• Use to promote granulation. • Use to manage pain. • Don't use when copious drainage is present.	• Use for autolytic debridement. • Use for primary dressing after revascularization. • Don't use on ischemic tissue.	• Use to protect the skin. • Use to promote epithelialization. • Don't use when copious drainage is present. • Don't use when cellulitis is present.
Hydrogel	• Don't use when copious drainage is present.	• Use to maintain a moist wound bed. • Use to debride.	• Use to manage pain. • Use to debride.
Transparent films	• Not indicated	• Use only after the ulcer is almost completely healed.	• Use to protect fragile skin. • Don't use when cellulitis is present.

• Be sure to choose the proper dressing for each ulcer. Remember, dressing choice depends on the characteristics of the ulcer as well as the ulcer type. (See *Dressings for vascular ulcers*.)

• For the most part, the wound care axiom of keeping dry tissues dry and moist tissues moist applies to vascular wounds. The one exception is an arterial ulcer, which must be kept dry until the area is revascularized. Then the axiom applies here as well.

• Whenever possible, avoid using tape on the patient's skin. Skin affected by vascular disease is fragile and new ulcers form easily.

Patient education

For the most part, the success or failure of treatment is in the patient's hands because he has the primary responsibility for caring for this chronic condition. A motivated patient is more likely to adhere to the treatment regimen — a fact you should keep in mind as you prepare patient-teaching sessions. Patient teaching should provide clear instructions and rationales to encourage active patient participation.

Patient participation

Pass these tips along to your patient to promote vascular ulcer healing and reduce his risk of developing new ulcers:

• Look at your skin every day. Use lotion on dry, flaky skin.
• Use your calf muscles! Frequent walks aid healing.
• Flex your feet up and down (as if you were using the gas pedal in the car) frequently when sitting.
• Elevate your legs whenever you sit.
• Wear shoes that fit well, and always wear socks under shoes.
• Wear your compression stockings as directed.
• Don't sit or stand for long periods of time.
• Strive to maintain the agreed upon target weight.
• Report any skin injury to your doctor.
• Don't smoke.

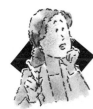

Quick quiz

1. Venous insufficiency can result from all of the following except:

    A.   venous hypertension.
    B.   venous thrombi.
    C.   edema.
    D.   vasoconstriction.

Answer: D. Vasoconstriction isn't a precipitating factor in venous insufficiency.

2. Your patient has venous insufficiency. His leg edema is best treated by:

    A.   compression and leg elevation.
    B.   diuretics and compression.
    C.   leg elevation and diuretics.
    D.   restricting fluid intake and compression.

Answer: A. Compression helps to manage edema when the patient is upright. Leg elevation uses gravity to maximize venous return.

3. ABI is:

    A.   a guide to venous hypertension.
    B.   a value that reflects the amount of blood flow to the ankle.
    C.   obtained in a sitting position with feet flat.
    D.   normal if it's above 0.5 mm Hg.

Answer: B. In ABI, each value reflects the ratio of ankle systolic pressure to brachial systolic pressure.

4. The best dressing type for an ischemic ulcer on the toe is:

    A.   hydrocolloid.
    B.   wet to dry.
    C.   dry.
    D.   hydrogel.

Answer: C. An ischemic — or arterial — ulcer should be kept dry until blood flow to the area is restored.

5. Which of the following signs or symptoms is a key indication of progressive arterial insufficiency?

    A.   Cyanosis when the foot is in a dependent position
    B.   Pain
    C.   Edema
    D.   Hyperpigmentation of the skin

Answer: B. Pain is the most common presenting symptom in arterial disease with or without an ulcer.

Scoring

✩✩✩   If you answered all five questions correctly, set off the fireworks! You deserve a splendid evening off tonight.

✩✩   If you answered three or four questions correctly, rock around the clock. You're dancing right through these quizzes.

✩   If you answered fewer than three questions correctly, don't look so glum. We're certain that your condition isn't chronic!

6

Pressure ulcers

Just the facts

In this chapter, you'll learn:

♦ causes of pressure ulcers

♦ factors that increase pressure ulcer risk and ways to detect them

♦ ways to prevent pressure ulcers

♦ pressure ulcer assessment and staging criteria

♦ treatment options.

A look at pressure ulcers

Pressure ulcers are a serious health problem. Although incidence figures vary widely because of differences in methodology, setting, and subjects, data gathered through 10 years of nationwide studies reveal that 10% to 15% of the general population suffer from chronic pressure ulcers. Although this finding is significant in itself, prevalence in some groups — such as patients with spinal cord injuries, patients in intensive care units, and nursing home residents — is shockingly higher.

At what cost?

Although prevalence statistics vary, what's become starkly evident are the costs associated with pressure ulcers — the cost in terms of suffering and diminished quality of life for patients, the cost to the health care industry in terms of resources consumed and manpower hours dedicated to managing the problem, and the very real monetary cost to individuals, health insurers, and government agencies.

The problem is so acute that many insurers and government agencies now track outcomes to discern whether specific interventions help treat pressure ulcers and to encourage prevention, early intervention, and closer monitoring by the health care industry. Because pressure ulcers are chronic conditions — they're hard

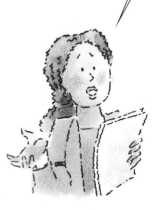

Pressure ulcers are problems for everyone. Not only do patients suffer from reduced quality of life but health insurers and government agencies also pay the price.

to heal and tend to recur frequently — prevention and early intervention are critical for more effective management.

Island OASIS

Data collected from Outcome and Assessment Information Set (OASIS) forms provide a basis for relating these costs to clinical outcomes. The OASIS-B1 form is currently used by home health care agencies, as mandated by the Centers for Medicare and Medicaid Services. (For more information, see the appendix Using the OASIS-B1 form.)

The closer you get

Better disease management in pressure ulcer cases depends on closer collaboration among government agencies, insurers, and health care professionals. There's heartening evidence that this group effort is developing. All involved are paying closer attention to prevention and the effectiveness of interventions, and they're finding better methods of quantifying and disseminating results. Soon, pressure ulcers will be a reportable condition for the Centers for Disease Control and Prevention. In addition, the health care objectives for the nation as a whole reflect a better understanding of the problem's severity. Healthy People 2010 (a report of the nation's near-term health care goals) includes a goal of reducing by 50% the prevalence of pressure ulcers in nursing home residents.

Healthy People 2010 takes a preventive approach to the nation's health care goals. Among these goals is a 50% reduction in pressure ulcers among nursing home residents.

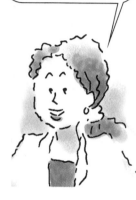

Causes

Chronic wounds are those that fail to heal in a timely manner, resist treatment, and tend to recur. Pressure ulcers are chronic wounds resulting from tissue death due to prolonged, irreversible ischemia brought on by compression of soft tissue.

All of us cells get the oxygen and nutrients we need from circulating blood.

When that blood flow is cut off, ischemia can result.

If you want to get technical

Technically speaking, pressure ulcers are the clinical manifestation of localized tissue death due to lack of blood flow in areas under pressure.

Simplify, simplify!

Now, let's back up a bit to break down and better understand this description. First of all, different tissues have different tolerances for compression. Muscle and fat have comparatively low tolerances for pressure, whereas skin has a somewhat higher tolerance. All cells, regardless of tissue type, depend on blood circulation for the oxygen and nutrients they need. Tissue compression interferes with circulation, reducing or completely cutting off blood flow. The result, known as *ischemia*, is that cells fail to receive adequate supplies of oxygen and nutrients. Unless the pressure relents, cells eventually die. By the time inflammation signals impending necrosis on the surface of the skin, it's likely that necrosis has occurred in deeper tissues.

Location, location, location

Pressure ulcers are most common in areas where pressure compresses soft tissue over a bony prominence in the body—the tissue is pinched between the outer pressure and the hard underlying surface. Other factors that contribute to the problem include shear, friction, and moisture. Planning effective interventions for prevention and treatment requires a sound understanding of the etiology of pressure ulcers.

Pressure

Capillaries are connected to arteries and veins through intermediary vessels called *arterioles* and *venules*. In healthy individuals, capillary filling pressure is approximately 32 mm Hg where arterioles connect to capillaries and 12 mm Hg where capillaries connect to venules. Therefore, external pressure greater than capillary filling pressure can cause problems. In frail or ill people, capillary filling pressures may be much lower. External pressure that exceeds capillary perfusion pressure compresses blood vessels and causes ischemia in the tissues supplied by those vessels.

Tip of the iceberg

If the pressure continues long enough, capillaries collapse and thrombose, toxic metabolic by-products accumulate, and cells in nearby muscle and subcutaneous tissues begin to die. Muscle and fat are less tolerant of interruptions in blood flow than skin. Consequently, by the time signs of impending necrosis appear on the skin, underlying tissue has probably suffered substantial damage. Keep this "tip of the iceberg" effect in mind when assessing the size of a pressure ulcer.

The pressure mounts

When external pressure exceeds venous capillary refill pressure (about 12 mm Hg), capillaries begin to leak. The resulting edema increases the amount of pressure on blood vessels, further impeding circulation. When interstitial pressure surpasses arterial intravascular pressure, blood is forced into nearby tissues (nonblanchable erythema). Continued capillary occlusion, lack of oxygen and nutri-

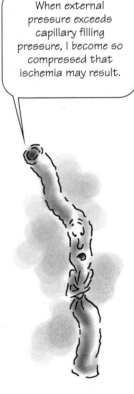

When external pressure exceeds capillary filling pressure, I become so compressed that ischemia may result.

Pressure points

Pressure points are likely areas for ulcer formation. These illustrations show the areas at highest risk for ulcers when the patient is in different positions.

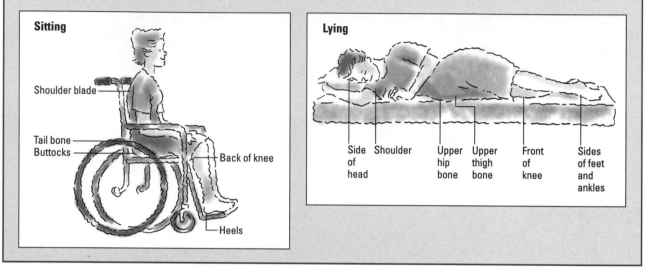

Sitting

Shoulder blade

Tail bone
Buttocks

Back of knee

Heels

Lying

Side of head   Shoulder   Upper hip bone   Upper thigh bone   Front of knee   Sides of feet and ankles

ents, and buildup of toxic waste leads to necrosis of muscle, subcutaneous tissue and, ultimately, the dermis and epidermis.

Spreading the load

The force associated with any given pressure increases as the amount of body surface exposed to the pressure decreases. For example, the force exerted on the buttocks of a person lying in bed is about 70 mm Hg. However, when the same person sits on a hard surface, the force exerted on the ischial tuberosities can be as much as 300 mm Hg. Consequently, bony prominences are particularly susceptible to pressure ulcers. However, they aren't the only areas at risk. Ulcers can develop on any soft tissue subjected to prolonged pressure. (See *Pressure points*.)

Between a bone and a hard place

When blood vessels, muscle, subcutaneous fat, and skin are compressed between a bone and an external surface—a bed or chair, for instance—pressure is exerted on the tissues from both the external surface and the bone. In effect, the external surface produces pressure and the bone produces counterpressure. These opposing forces create a cone-shaped pressure gradient. (See *Understanding the pressure gradient*.) Although the pressure affects all tissues between these two points, tissues closest to the bony prominence suffer the greatest damage.

Understanding the pressure gradient

In the illustration at right, the V-shaped pressure gradient results from the upward force exerted by the supporting surface and the downward force of the bony prominence. Pressure is greatest on tissues at the apex of the gradient and lessens to the right and left of this point.

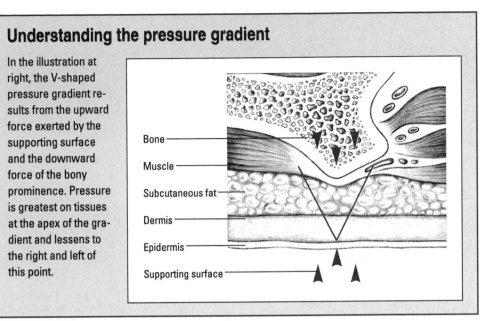

Bone

Muscle

Subcutaneous fat

Dermis

Epidermis

Supporting surface

Under pressure

Over time, pressure causes a growing discomfort that prompts a person to change position before tissue ischemia occurs. In ulcer formation, an inverse relationship exists between time and pressure. Typically, low pressure for long periods is far more damaging than high pressure for short periods. For example, a pressure of 70 mm Hg sustained for 2 hours or longer almost always causes irreversible tissue damage, whereas a pressure of 240 mm Hg can be endured for a short time with little or no tissue damage. Furthermore, after the time-pressure threshold for damage passes, damage continues even after the pressure stops. Although pressure ulcers can result from one period of sustained pressure, they're more likely to result from repeated ischemic events without adequate intervening time for recovery.

Shear

Shearing force intensifies the pressure's destructive effects. Shear is a mechanical force that runs parallel, rather than perpendicular, to an area of skin; deep tissues feel the brunt of the force.

The shear truth of it

Shearing force is most likely to develop during repositioning or when a patient slides down after being placed in high Fowler's position. However, simply elevating the head of the bed increases

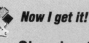

Now I get it!

Shearing force

Shear is a mechanical force parallel, rather than perpendicular, to an area of tissue. In the illustration at right, gravity pulls the body down the incline of the bed. The skeleton and attached tissues move, but the skin remains stationary, held in place by friction between the skin and the bed linen. The skeleton and attached tissues actually slide within the skin, causing skin to pucker in the gluteal area.

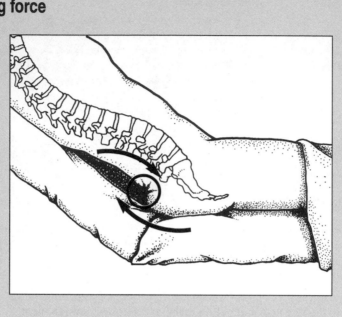

Keep in mind that elderly patients and patients who have spastic conditions or wear appliances are at increased risk for friction injuries.

shear and pressure in the sacral and coccygeal areas; gravity pulls the body down but the skin on the back resists the motion because of friction between the skin and the sheets. The result is that the skeleton (and attached tissues) actually slides somewhat beneath the skin (evidenced by the puckering of skin in the gluteal area), generating shearing force between outer layers of tissue and deeper layers. The force generated is enough to obstruct, tear, or stretch blood vessels (See *Shearing force*).

Shearing force reduces the length of time that tissue can endure a given pressure before ischemia or necrosis occurs. A sufficiently high level of shearing force can halve the amount of pressure needed to produce vascular occlusion. Research indicates that shearing force is responsible for the high incidence of triangular shaped sacral ulcers and the large areas of tunneling or deep sinus tracts beneath these ulcers.

Friction

Friction is another potentially damaging mechanical force. Friction develops as one surface moves across another surface — for example, the patient's skin sliding across the bed sheet. Abrasions are wounds created by friction.

Those at particularly high risk for tissue damage due to friction include patients who have uncontrollable movements or spastic conditions, patients who wear braces or appliances that rub against the skin, and older patients. Friction is also a problem for patients who have trouble lifting themselves during repositioning. Rubbing against the sheet can result in an abrasion, which increases the potential for deeper tissue damage. Elevating the head of the bed, as discussed earlier, generates friction between the patient's skin and the bed linen as gravity tugs the patient's body downward. As the skeleton moves inside the skin, friction and shearing force combine to increase the risk of tissue damage in the sacral area. Such dry lubricants as cornstarch and adherent dressings with slippery backings can help reduce the impact of friction.

Excessive moisture

Prolonged exposure to moisture can waterlog, or macerate, skin. Maceration contributes to pressure ulcer formation by softening the connective tissue. Macerated epidermis erodes more easily, degenerates, and eventually sloughs off. In addition, damp skin adheres to bed linen more readily, making friction's effects more profound. Consequently, moist skin is five times more likely to develop ulcers than dry skin. Excessive moisture can result from perspiration, wound drainage, bathing, or fecal or urinary incontinence.

Risk factors

Factors that increase the risk of developing pressure ulcers include advancing age, immobility, incontinence, infection, poor nutrition, and low blood pressure. High-risk patients, whether in an institution or at home, should be assessed regularly for pressure ulcers.

Age

With advancing age, the skin becomes more fragile as epidermal turnover slows, vascularization decreases, and skin layers adhere less securely to one another. Older adults have less lean body mass and less subcutaneous tissue cushioning bony areas. Consequently, they're more likely to suffer tissue damage due to friction, shear, and pressure. Other common problems include poor nutrition, poor hydration, and impaired respiratory or immune systems.

Immobility

Immobility may be the greatest risk factor for pressure ulcer development. The patient's ability to move in response to pressure sensations as well as the frequency with which his position is changed should always be considered in risk assessment.

Incontinence

Incontinence increases a patient's exposure to moisture and, over time, increases his risk of skin breakdown. Both urinary and fecal incontinence create problems as a result of excessive moisture and chemical irritation. Due to pathogens in the stool, fecal incontinence can cause more skin damage than urinary incontinence.

Infection

Although the role of infection in pressure ulceration isn't fully understood, animal studies on the effects of pressure and infection indicate that compression encourages a localized increase in bacteria concentration. Bacteria injected into animals localized at the compression site, resulting in necrosis at lower pressures relative to the control group. Researchers concluded that compressed skin lowers local resistance to bacterial infection and that infection may reduce the pressure needed to cause tissue necrosis. Furthermore, researchers noted higher infection rates in pedicle flaps when denervation or loss of motor and sensory nerve function occurred. This may explain why neurologically impaired patients are more susceptible to infection and pressure ulceration.

Nutrition

Proper nutrition is vitally important to tissue integrity. A strong correlation exists between poor nutrition and pressure ulceration, yet nutrition is all too commonly overlooked during treatment.

Albumin acumen

Increased protein is required for the body to heal itself. Albumin is one of the key proteins in the body. A patient's serum albumin lev-

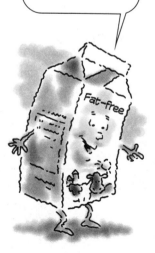

Adequate nutritional intake, particularly of dietary proteins, is an important part of maintaining tissue integrity and preventing ulcers.

el is an important indicator of his protein levels. A subnormal serum albumin level is a late manifestation of protein deficiency. Normal serum albumin levels range from 3.5 to 5.0 g/dl. Serum albumin deficits are ranked as follows:

- mild — 3.0 to 3.5 g/dl
- moderate — 2.5 to 3.0 g/dl
- severe — less than 2.5 g/dl.

Pressure ulcer occurrence and severity are linked to malnutrition. One recent study found a direct correlation between pressure ulcer stage and degree of hypoalbuminemia (serum albumin level below 3.5 g/dl). Monitor the serum albumin levels of a high-risk patient and plan on nutritional intervention if he has hypoproteinemia.

Blood pressure

Low arterial blood pressure is clearly linked to tissue ischemia, particularly in vascular patients. When blood pressure is low, the body shunts blood away from the peripheral vascular system that serves the skin and toward vital organs to ensure their health. As perfusion drops, the skin is less tolerant of sustained external pressure, and the risk of damage due to ischemia rises.

Risk factor assessment

Several assessment tools are available to help determine a patient's risk of pressure ulcers. Most are based on the work of Doreen Norton, who studied the pressure ulcer problem in Great Britain. Some years later, Gosnell and Braden developed a more refined scale based on data from independent studies.

Common denominators

Most scales use the following factors to determine a patient's risk of developing pressure ulcers:

- immobility
- inactivity
- incontinence
- malnutrition
- impaired mental status or sensation.

Each category receives a value based on the patient's condition. The sum of these values determines the patient's score and level of risk. Scores for each category as well as the assessment as a whole help the care team develop appropriate interventions. Most health care facilities require an assessment score for every patient admitted. The Agency for Health Care Policy and Research

Memory jogger

To remember the five factors commonly used to determine a patient's risk of developing pressure ulcers, think of the 5 **I's:**

Immobility

Inactivity

Incontinence

Improper nutrition (malnutrition)

Impaired mental status or sensation.

Guidelines for Pressure Ulcer Prediction and Prevention recommends use of either the Norton or Braden scale.

The Braden scale

The Braden Pressure Sore Risk Assessment Scale is the most widely used scale. This tool scores etiologic factors that contribute to prolonged pressure as well as factors that contribute to diminished tissue tolerance for pressure. Factors scored in this assessment include sensory perception, moisture, activity, mobility, nutrition, and friction and shear. (See *Braden scale: Predicting pressure ulcer risk*, pages 136 and 137.) Each factor receives a score of 1 to 4, with the exception of friction and shear, which receives a score of 1 to 3. The highest possible score is 23; the lower the score, the higher the patient's risk of pressure ulceration. A score of 18 or lower denotes a risk of pressure ulcers.

In nursing home populations, most pressure ulcers develop during the 2 weeks immediately following admission, so early identification of at-risk patients is crucial. No definitive guidelines exist for how often to reassess a patient; however, a common-sense approach would be to reassess the patient when his condition changes or in the event that he becomes chair-bound or bedridden.

Prevention

Pressure ulcer prevention focuses on compensating for prevailing risk factors and addressing the underlying pathophysiology. When planning interventions, be sure to adopt a holistic approach and consider all of the patient's needs.

Managing pressure

Managing the intensity and duration of pressure is a fundamental goal in prevention, especially for patients with mobility limitations. Frequent, careful repositioning helps the patient avoid the damaging repetitive pressure that can cause tissue ischemia and subsequent necrosis. When repositioning the patient, it's important to reduce the duration and the intensity of pressure.

Positioning

Anytime that you reposition the patient, look for telltale areas of reddened skin and make sure the new position doesn't place weight on these areas. Avoid the use of donut-shaped supports or ring cushions that encircle the ischemic area because these can reduce blood flow to an even wider expanse of tissue. If the affected area is on an extremity, use pillows to support the limb and reduce pressure. As noted earlier, avoid raising the head of the bed more than 30 degrees to prevent tissue damage due to friction and shearing force.

Short stepping it

Inactivity increases a patient's risk of ulcer development. To the degree that the patient is physically able, encourage activity. Start with a short step—help him out of bed and into a chair. As his tolerance improves, help him walk around the room and then down the hall.

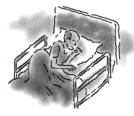

Positioning a patient in bed

When the patient is on his side, never allow weight to rest directly on the greater trochanter of the femur. Instead, have the patient rest his weight on his buttock and use a pillow or foam wedge to maintain the position. This position ensures that no pressure is placed on the trochanter or sacrum. Also, a pillow placed between the knees or ankles minimizes the pressure exerted when one limb lies atop the other. (See *Repositioning a reclining patient*, page 138.)

Heel appeal

Heels present a particularly difficult challenge. Even with the aid of specially designed cushions, reducing the pressure on heels to below capillary refill pressure is almost impossible. Instead, suspend the patient's foot so the bony prominence on the heel is under no pressure. A pillow or foam cushion under the patient's calves can permit a comfortable position while suspending the foot. Take care to avoid knee contraction, however.

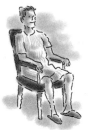

Positioning a seated patient

Unlikely as it seems, a patient is more likely to develop pressure ulcers from sitting than from reclining. Sitting tends to focus all of the patient's weight on the relatively small surface areas of the buttocks, thighs, and soles. Much of this weight is focused on the small area of tissue covering the ischial tuberosities. Proper posture and alignment help ensure that the weight of the patient's body is distributed as evenly as possible.

Proper posture when sitting is a key part of pressure ulcer prevention. It looks like you're doing a good job keeping your back straight, knees comfortably parted, and feet flat.

In the key of posture

Proper posture alone can significantly reduce the patient's risk of ulcers at the ankles, elbows, forearms, wrists, and knees. Explain proper posture to your patient, if necessary, as described here:
• Sit with back erect and against the back of the chair, thighs parallel to the floor, knees comfortably parted, and

(Text continues on page 138.)

Braden scale: Predicting pressure ulcer risk

The Braden scale, shown here, is the most reliable of several existing instruments for assessing a patient's risk of developing pressure ulcers. The lower the score, the greater the risk.

Patient's name _____ *Kevin Lawson* _____ Evaluator's name _____ *Joan Norris, RN* _____

SENSORY PERCEPTION Ability to respond meaningfully to pressure-related discomfort	**1. Completely limited:** Unresponsive (doesn't moan, flinch, or grasp) to painful stimuli because of diminished level of consciousness or sedation OR Limited ability to feel pain over most of body surface	**2. Very limited:** Responds only to painful stimuli; can't communicate discomfort except by moaning or restlessness OR Has a sensory impairment that limits the ability to feel pain or discomfort over one-half of body
MOISTURE Degree to which skin is exposed to moisture	**1. Constantly moist:** Skin is kept moist almost constantly by perspiration, urine, etc.; dampness is detected every time patient is moved or turned	**2. Very moist:** Skin is often but not always moist; linen must be changed at least once per shift
ACTIVITY Degree of physical activity	**1. Bedfast:** Confined to bed	**2. Chairfast:** Ability to walk severely limited or nonexistent; can't bear own weight or must be assisted into chair or wheelchair
MOBILITY Ability to change and control body position	**1. Completely immobile:** Doesn't make even slight changes in body or extremity position without assistance	**2. Very limited:** Makes occasional slight changes in body or extremity position but can't make frequent or significant changes independently
NUTRITION Usual food intake pattern	**1. Very poor:** Never eats a complete meal; rarely eats more than one-third of any food offered; eats two servings or less of protein (meat or dairy products) per day; takes fluids poorly; doesn't take a liquid dietary supplement OR Is NPO or maintained on clear liquids or I.V. fluids for more than 5 days	**2. Probably inadequate:** Rarely eats a complete meal and generally eats only about one-half of any food offered; protein intake includes only three servings of meat or dairy products per day; occasionally takes a dietary supplement OR Receives less than optimum amount of liquid diet or tube feeding
FRICTION AND SHEAR	**1. Problem:** Requires moderate to maximum assistance in moving; complete lifting without sliding against sheets is impossible; frequently slides down in bed or chair, requiring frequent repositioning with maximum assistance; spasticity, contractures, or agitation leads to almost constant friction	**2. Potential problem:** Moves feebly or requires minimum assistance; during a move, skin probably slides to some extent against sheets, chair restraints, or other devices; maintains relatively good position in chair or bed most of the time but occasionally slides down

Date of assessment _____ 3/21/03 _____

3. Slightly limited: Responds to verbal commands but can't always communicate discomfort or need to be turned OR Has some sensory impairment that limits ability to feel pain or discomfort in one or two extremities	**4. No impairment:** Responds to verbal commands; has no sensory deficit that would limit ability to feel or voice pain or discomfort	3
3. Occasionally moist: Skin is occasionally moist, requiring an extra linen change approximately once per day	**4. Rarely moist:** Skin is usually dry; linen only requires changing at routine intervals	3
3. Walks occasionally: Walks occasionally during day, but for very short distances, with or without assistance; spends most of each shift in bed or chair	**4. Walks frequently:** Walks outside the room at least twice per day and inside room at least once every 2 hours during waking hours	4
3. Slightly limited: Makes frequent though slight changes in body or extremity position independently	**4. No limitations:** Makes major and frequent changes in position without assistance	4
3. Adequate: Eats over one-half of most meals; eats four servings of protein (meat, dairy products) each day; occasionally refuses a meal, but usually takes a supplement if offered OR Is on a tube feeding or TPN regimen that probably meets most nutritional needs	**4. Excellent:** Eats most of every meal and never refuses a meal; usually eats four or more servings of meat and dairy products; occasionally eats between meals; doesn't require supplementation	4
3. No apparent problem: Moves in bed and in chair independently and has sufficient muscle strength to lift up completely during move; maintains good position in bed or chair at all times		3
	TOTAL SCORE	21

Repositioning a reclining patient

When repositioning a reclining patient, use the Rule of 30—that is, raise the head of the bed 30 degrees (as shown at right). Avoid raising the head of the bed more than 30 degrees to prevent the buildup of shearing pressure. When you must raise it more—at meal times, for instance—keep the periods brief.

As you reposition the patient from his left side to his right side, make sure his weight rests on his buttock, not his hip bone. This reduces pressure on the trochanter and sacrum. The angle between the bed and an imaginary lateral line through his hips should be about 30 degrees. If needed, use pillows or a foam wedge to help the patient maintain the proper position (see illustration at right). Cushion pressure points, such as the knees or shoulders, with pillows as well.

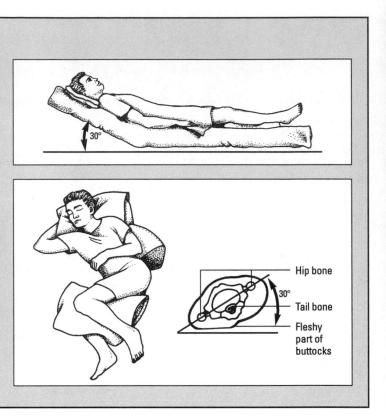

arms horizontal and supported by the arms of the chair. This posture distributes weight evenly over the available body surface area.

• Keep feet flat on the floor to protect the heels from focused pressure and distribute the weight of the legs over the largest available surface area—the soles.

• Avoid slouching, which causes shearing force and friction and places undue pressure on the sacrum and coccyx.

• Keep the thighs and arms parallel to ensure that weight is evenly distributed all along the thighs and forearms, instead of being focused on the ischial tuberosities and elbows, respectively.

• Part the knees to keep knees and ankles from rubbing together.

The comforts of home

If the patient likes to use an ottoman or footstool, check to see if his knees end up above the level of his hips. If so, it means that his weight has shifted from the back of his thighs to the ischial tuberosities—and that he needs to find a different footstool. The same problem—knees above hips—can occur if the chair itself is too short for the patient.

Patients at risk should reposition themselves every 15 minutes while sitting, if they can. Patients with spinal cord injuries can perform wheelchair pushups to intermittently relieve pressure on the buttocks and sacrum. This requires a fair amount of upper body strength, however, and some patients might not have the strength. Others may have injuries that preclude using this technique.

Support aids and cushions

Pillows may be the most enduring support tools on the planet, but they're no longer the only options available. Today, people can choose from a vast array of support surfaces and cushioning aids. Special beds, mattresses, and seating options that employ foams, gels, water, and air as cushioning agents make it possible to tailor a comprehensive and personal system of supports for your patient.

A pillow is always good for support but it isn't your only option.

Effective care depends on knowledge of the classes and types of products. In the course of your work, take time to learn as much as you can about these products. (See *Pressure reduction devices*, page 140.)

False security

Be informed, but be cautious as well. Using these devices can instill a false sense of security. It's important to remember that as helpful as these devices may be, they aren't substitutes for attentive care. Patients require individual turning schedules regardless of the equipment used, and this schedule depends on your assessment of the patient's tolerance for pressure.

Beds and mattresses

When we discuss horizontal support surfaces we are, for the most part, talking about beds, mattresses, and mattress overlays. These products employ foams, gels, water, and air to minimize the pressure a patient experiences while lying in bed.

Beds

Specialty beds, such as oscillating and turning beds, relieve pressure by turning the patient or help lift the patient to reduce the risk of friction and shear. However, they're expensive and are rarely an option for a patient returning home.

Mattresses

Most mattresses worth considering use some form or manipulation of foam, gel, air, or water to cushion the patient. Foam core

Pressure reduction devices

Here are some special pads, mattresses, and beds that help relieve pressure when a patient is confined to one position for long periods.

Gel pads
Gel pads disperse pressure over a wide surface area.

Water mattress or pads
A wave effect provides even distribution of body weight.

Alternating-pressure air mattress
Alternating deflation and inflation of mattress tubes changes areas of pressure.

Foam mattress or pads
Foam areas, which must be at least 3″ to 4″ (7.5- to 10-cm) thick, cushion skin, minimizing pressure.

Low-air-loss beds
This bed surface consists of inflated air cushions. Each section is adjusted for optimal pressure relief for the patient's body size.

Air-fluidized bed
An air-fluidized bed contains beads that move under an airflow to support the patient, thus reducing shearing force and friction.

Stryker or Foster frame or CircOlectric bed
These devices relieve pressure by turning the patient.

Mechanical lifting devices
Lift sheets and other mechanical lifting devices prevent shearing by lifting the patient rather than dragging him across the bed.

Padding
Pillows, towels, and soft blankets can reduce pressure in body hollows.

Foot cradle
A foot cradle lifts the bed linens to relieve pressure over the feet.

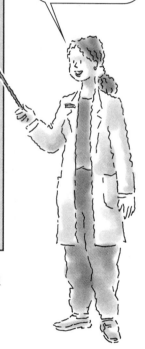

The more you learn about available options, the better prepared you are to best care for your patient.

mattresses can provide the same benefits derived from a standard mattress with a foam overlay. Low-air-loss and high-air-loss mattresses are specialized support devices that pass air over the patient's skin. These mattresses promote evaporation and are especially useful when skin maceration is a problem.

Water works

Water mattresses and some air mattresses use different media, but similar techniques, to evenly distribute pressure under the patient. Water mattresses use gentle wave motion to maintain even distribution of pressure, whereas several types of air mattress alternately inflate and deflate tubes within the mattress to distribute pressure.

Mattress overlays

The most common mattress overlays used in pressure ulcer prevention are foam, air, and gel overlays. Foam overlays should be at least 3″ (7.6 cm) thick for the average patient; thicker is even better. Although 2″ (5.1 cm) foam overlays may add comfort, they aren't suitable for patients at risk for pressure ulcers. Solid foam is preferable to the convoluted version. Be sure to select an overlay constructed from higher-quality foam because it will last longer.

Palm reading

If the patient's weight completely compresses a mattress overlay, the overlay isn't helping. To make sure the patient isn't bottoming out, hand check whenever a new overlay is put into service or if you suspect an overlay is breaking down. To hand check an overlay, slide one hand — palm up and fingers outstretched — between the mattress overlay and the mattress. If you can feel the patient's body through the overlay, replace the overlay with a thicker one or add more air to the mattress.

Support aids for sitting

Products designed to help prevent pressure ulcers while sitting fall into two broad categories: products that relieve pressure and products that ease repositioning.

Ambulatory and wheelchair-dependent patients should use seat cushions to distribute weight over the largest possible surface area. Wheelchair-dependent patients require an especially rugged seat cushion that can stand up to the rigors of daily use. In most instances, a good foam cushion 3″ to 4″ (7.5 to 10 cm) thick suffices. However, many wheelchair-seating clinics now use computers to create custom seating systems tailored to fit the physiology and needs of each patient. For patients with spinal cord injuries, the selection of wheelchair seating is based on pressure evaluation, lifestyle, postural stability, continence, and cost. Custom seats and cushions are more expensive; however, in this case, the added expense is justifiable. Encourage wheelchair patients to replace seat cushions as soon as their current one begins to deteriorate.

A position on repositioning

Repositioning is just as important when the patient is sitting as when he's reclining. For a patient requiring assistance, various devices are available. Such devices as overhead frames, trapezes, walkers, and canes can help the patient reposition himself as necessary. Health care personnel can help maneuver I.V. poles and other support equipment.

Managing skin integrity

An effective skin integrity management plan includes regular inspections for tissue breakdown, routine cleaning and moisturizing, and steps to protect the skin from incontinence, if this is an issue.

Inspecting the skin

The patient's skin should be routinely inspected for pressure areas, depending on the patient's assessed risk and his ability to tolerate pressure. Check for pallor and areas of redness — both signs of ischemia. Be aware that redness that occurs after the pressure is removed (called *reactive hyperemia*) is commonly the first external sign of ischemia due to pressure.

> Cleaning the skin with mild soap and warm water and patting the skin dry help to maintain skin integrity.

Cleaning the skin

Usually, cleaning with a gentle soap and warm water suffices for daily skin hygiene. Use a soft cloth to pat, rather than rub, the skin dry. Avoid scrubbing or the use of harsh cleaning agents.

Moisturizing the skin

Skin becomes dry, flaky, and less pliable when it loses moisture. Dry skin is more susceptible to ulceration. The number of skin moisturizing products available is truly staggering, so it shouldn't be hard to find one that the patient likes. The three categories of skin moisturizers are lotions, creams, and ointments.

Lotion notion

Lotions are dissolved powder crystals held in suspension by surfactants. Lotions have the highest water content and evaporate faster than any other type of moisturizer. Consequently, lotions must be applied more often. The high water content is why lotions feel cool as they're applied.

Cream regime

Creams are preparations of oil and water; they're more occlusive than lotions. Creams don't have to be applied as often as lotions; three or four applications per day should do the trick. Creams are better for preventing moisture loss due to evaporation than for replenishing skin moisture.

Ointment appointment

Ointments are preparations of water in oil (typically lanolin or petrolatum). They're the most occlusive and longest lasting form of moisturizer. Studies indicate that petrolatum is a more effective moisturizer than lanolin.

Protecting the skin

Although some moisture is good, too much is a problem. Waterlogged skin is easily eroded by friction and is more susceptible to irritants and bacteria colonization than dry skin. Close monitoring helps head off problems before they escalate.

Skin protection is particularly important if the patient is incontinent. Urine and feces introduce chemical irritants and bacteria as well as moisture, which can speed skin breakdown. To effectively manage incontinence, first determine the cause and then plan interventions that protect skin integrity while addressing the underlying problem.

In older adults, don't assume that incontinence is a normal part of aging. It isn't. Instead, consider factors that can precipitate incontinence, such as:
- fecal impaction and tube feeding (can cause diarrhea)
- a reaction to medication (can cause urinary incontinence)
- urinary tract infection
- mobility problems (can keep the patient from reaching the bathroom in time)
- confusion or embarrassment (can keep the patient from asking for a bedpan or help getting to the bathroom).

Lend a helping hand

Whether the underlying cause is reversible or not, encourage the patient to ask for help when he needs a bedpan or needs to go to the bathroom. Use incontinence collectors, diapers or underpads, and skin barriers as appropriate to minimize skin damage. (See *Managing incontinence*, page 144.) Step up the frequency of inspections, cleansing, and moisturizing for these patients.

Managing nutrition

Proper nutrition is essential to both ulcer prevention and healing.

Dietary intake

Protein is particularly important to skin maintenance. Your patient needs a balanced diet that includes approximately 0.8 g/kg/day of protein. For most healthy adults, this means eating one or two 3-ounce servings of protein each day in the form of meat, milk, cheese, or eggs.

Body weight

Low body weight is a problem for many pressure ulcer patients. An underlying illness or anorexia can make eating undesirable or impossible. To head off problems and to monitor the results of nutritional interventions, weigh the patient weekly. If the patient history includes an unintentional weight loss of 10 lb (4.5 kg) or more during the previous 6 months, malnutrition may be the cause.

Weigh your patient weekly to prevent problems associated with low body weight and to monitor the results of nutritional interventions.

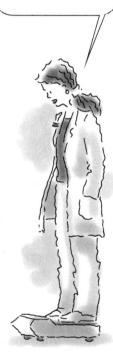

Managing incontinence

Incontinent patients require careful monitoring and special interventions to prevent skin damage caused by excessive moisture, chemical irritation, or microbial infection. Three types of aids can help you manage incontinence and minimize its impact on your patient: incontinence collectors, incontinence diapers and underpads, and topical barriers.

Incontinence collectors
• Condom catheters can help manage urinary incontinence in men (similar but less effective devices exist for women).
• Fecal incontinence collectors are pectin skin barriers with an attached, drainable pouch (similar to colostomy pouching systems).
• Collectors need to be changed on a regular schedule. Rectal tubes aren't a good alternative because they can cause such complications as vasovagal response or ischemia of anal tissue.

Incontinence diapers and underpads
• Diapers and underpads wick moisture away from the patient's skin. Underpads and diaper alternatives include disposable absorbent gel diapers, disposable cellulose core diapers, and laundered reusable cloth diapers.
• Studies indicate that disposable gel diapers are significantly more effective in reducing wetness and maintaining normal skin pH than other alternatives. Reusable cloth diapers offer the least expensive alternative.

• Don't be tempted to put a plastic or paper linen saver under an incontinent patient; this holds moisture next to the patient's skin and compounds the problem.
• Don't secure the pad to the patient. Underpads work by absorbing wetness and allowing air to circulate over the skin, drying it.
• Diapers and underpads require routine monitoring so they can be changed promptly after urination or voiding.

Topical skin barriers
• Liquid copolymer film barriers protect intact skin from the damaging effects of incontinence. They're available in aerosol form or as disposable wipes. As they dry, these products form a strong, almost plasticlike barrier on the skin's surface that isn't easily washed off during normal cleaning.
• Paste is an excellent skin barrier. A paste is an ointment that contains powder for thickness and durability. Many pastes contain zinc oxide. Pastes can be removed with mineral oil.

Pressure ulcer assessment

Pressure ulcers can occur even with the best preventive measures. Effective treatment depends on a thorough assessment of the developing wound. Meaningful ulcer assessment requires a systematic and objective approach. Clinical assessment should include:
• ulcer history, including etiology, duration, and prior treatment
• anatomic location
• stage
• size (length, width, depth in centimeters)
• sinus tracts, undermining, and tunneling
• drainage
• necrotic tissue (slough and eschar)
• granulation tissue (present or not)
• epithelialization (present or not).

On the border

Ulcer borders can provide clues to healing potential. Assess skin around the ulcer for:
- redness
- warmth
- induration or hardness
- swelling
- signs of infection.

Before you examine the ulcer, assess the patient's pain. In most cases, pressure ulcers cause some degree of pain; in some cases, pain is severe. Have the patient rate his pain on a visual analog scale of 0 to 10, with 0 representing no pain and 10 representing severe pain. Similarly, ask the patient whether the pain interferes with his ability to function normally and, if so, to what degree.

Location

Common locations for pressure ulcers include:
- sacrum
- coccyx
- ischial tuberosities
- greater trochanters
- elbows
- heels
- scapulae
- occipital bone
- sternum
- ribs
- iliac crests
- patellae
- lateral malleoli
- medial malleoli.

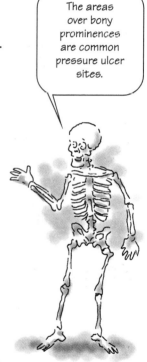

The areas over bony prominences are common pressure ulcer sites.

Bottoming out

Ulcers are more common on the lower half of the body because it has more major bony prominences and more body weight than the upper half of the body. Two-thirds of pressure ulcers occur within the pelvic girdle.

Characteristics

Tissue involvement ranges from blanchable erythema to the deep destruction of tissue associated with a full-thickness wound. Pressure against tissue interrupts blow flow and causes pallor due to tissue ischemia. If prolonged, ischemia causes irreversible and extensive tissue damage.

Reactive hyperemia

Usually, reactive hyperemia is the first visible sign of ischemia. When the pressure causing ischemia is released, skin flushes red as blood rushes back into the tissue. This reddening is called reactive hyperemia, and it's due to a protective mechanism in the body that dilates vessels in the affected area to increase the blood flow and speed oxygen to starved tissues. Reactive hyperemia first appears as a bright flush that lasts about one-half or three-quarters as long as the ischemic period. If the applied pressure is too high for too long, reactive hyperemia fails to meet the demand for blood and tissue damage occurs.

Blanchable erythema

Blanchable erythema (redness) can signal imminent tissue damage. Erythema results from capillary dilation near the skin's surface. In the patient with pressure ulcers, the redness results from the release of ischemia-causing pressure. Blanchable erythema is redness that blanches—turns white—when pressed with a fingertip and then immediately turns red again when pressure is removed. Tissue exhibiting blanchable erythema usually resumes its normal color within 24 hours and suffers no long-term damage. However, the longer it takes for tissue to recover from finger pressure, the higher the patient's risk of developing pressure ulcers.

In dark-skinned patients, erythema is hard to discern. Use bright light and look for taut, shiny patches of skin with a purplish tinge. Also, assess carefully for localized heat, induration, or edema, which can be better indicators of ischemia than erythema.

Nonblanchable erythema

Nonblanchable erythema can be the first sign of tissue destruction. In high-risk patients, nonblanchable tissue can develop in as little as 2 hours. The redness associated with nonblanchable erythema is more intense and doesn't change when compressed with a finger. If recognized and treated early, nonblanchable erythema is reversible.

What you can't see

In many cases, the full extent of ulceration can't be determined by visual inspection because there may be extensive undermining along fascial planes. For example, tunneling can connect ulcers over the sacrum to ulcers over the trochanter of the femur or the ischial tuberosities. These cavities can contain extensive necrotic tissue.

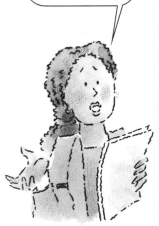

In many cases, the full extent of ulceration can't be determined by visual inspection because extensive undermining may exist along fascial planes.

Size

Using a disposable measuring tape, measure wound length (in centimeters) as the longest dimension of the wound and width as the longest distance perpendicular to the length. Alternatively, carefully trace the wound margins on a piece of paper. In addition, a growing number of facilities now use wound photography. Measure the ulcer's depth at its deepest point by inserting a gloved finger or a cotton-tipped swab. If you're using a probe other than your finger, be very careful; it's easy to cause further damage. Note any visible tunnels or undermining. If possible, use a gloved finger to gauge the extent.

Color

Wound color is a good indication of wound status. Record wound color using the red-yellow-black classification system. If more than one color is evident, classify the wound using the least healthy color.

Base

The type of tissue in the ulcer base determines the potential for healing and the type of treatment. Know how to identify necrotic tissue, granulation tissue, and epithelial tissue.

Necrotic tissue

Necrotic tissue may appear as a moist yellow or gray area of tissue that's separating from viable tissue. When dry, necrotic tissue appears as thick, hard, and leathery black eschar. Areas of necrotic or devitalized tissue may mask underlying abscesses and collections of fluid. Before the ulcer can begin to heal, necrotic tissue, drainage, and metabolic wastes must be removed from the wound.

Granulation tissue

Granulation tissue appears as beefy red, bumpy, shiny tissue in the base of the ulcer. As it heals, a full-thickness ulcer develops more and more granulation tissue. Such factors as tissue oxygenation, tissue hydration, and nutrition can alter the color and quality of granulation tissue.

Epithelial tissue

Epithelialization is the regeneration of epidermis across the ulcer surface. It appears as pale or dark pink skin, first becoming evident at ulcer borders in full-thickness wounds and as islands around hair follicles in partial-thickness wounds. Wound healing can be assessed and quantified by the percentage of surface covered by new epithelium.

Drainage

Ulcers with drainage, or exudate, take longer to heal. Drainage characteristics include amount, color, consistency, and odor. Record the amount as scant, moderate, large, or copious. Describe the color and consistency together with clear, descriptive terms, such as:
- serous — clear, watery
- serosanguinous — clear red or reddish brown
- purulent — thick, yellow, cloudy.

The nose knows

Odor is a subjective observation — one that can suggest infection. It's important to clean the wound thoroughly before assessing the color and odor of drainage. Otherwise, perceived drainage may be, in actuality, a combination of dressing residue and dead cells — a combination that always produces a noxious odor. However, putrid odor that remains after wound cleaning may indicate anaerobic infection.

Margins

Pressure ulcer edges have distinct characteristics, including color, thickness, and degree of attachment to the wound base.

Assess the epithelial rim as an integral part of the wound base. Ideally, there should be a free border of epithelial cells. These are the cells that proliferate and migrate across the wound bed during healing. When epidermis at the ulcer edges thickens and rolls under, it impairs migration of epithelial cells. In epiboly, the wound edges thicken and the pressure ulcer becomes chronic, with little or no evidence of new tissue growth.

Tunnel troubles

In undermining, which occurs when necrosis of subcutaneous fat or muscle occurs, a pocket extends beneath the skin at the ulcer's edge. Tunneling differs from undermining in that both ends of a tunnel emerge through the skin's surface. In many cases, a tunnel connects two otherwise distinct pressure ulcers and it may be necessary to open the tunnel before the ulcer can heal.

Sometimes full-thickness pressure ulcers form tracts along fascial planes. When extensive, external palpation is the only way to determine the direction and length of the tracts. If this is necessary, use a felt-tipped pen to outline the tract on the skin and measure the resulting image.

Surrounding skin

Assess intact skin surrounding the ulcer for redness, warmth, induration (hardness), swelling, and signs of infection. Palpate for heat, pain, and edema. The ulcer bed should be moist, but the surrounding skin should be dry. The skin should be adequately moisturized but neither macerated nor eroded. Macerated skin appears waterlogged and may turn white at the wound's edges.

A saline-soaked dressing can cause maceration of surrounding skin, unless the skin is protected. Other common causes of maceration include wound drainage and urine or feces contamination. Irritation or stripping may be the result of poor technique during dressing changes.

Keep your eye out for white, waterlogged skin around the wound's edges. This might indicate maceration.

Pressure ulcer staging

The most widely used system for staging pressure ulcers is the classification system developed by the National Pressure Ulcer Advisory Panel (NPUAP). This staging system, which defines four stages, has been adopted by the Agency for Health Care Policy and Research (AHCPR) Pressure Ulcer Guideline Panels and is published in both sets of AHCPR Clinical Practice Guidelines for Pressure Ulcers.

Now appearing on stage

Staging reflects the depth and extent of tissue involvement. Restaging isn't needed unless deeper layers of tissue are exposed by treatments such as debridement. Keep in mind that although staging is useful for classifying pressure ulcers, it's only one part of a comprehensive assessment. Ulcer characteristics and the condition of the surrounding skin provide equally important clues to the ulcer's prognosis.

Stage I

A stage I pressure ulcer is an area of skin with observable pressure-related changes when compared to an adjacent area or to the same region on the other side of the body. Indicators include a change in one or more of the following characteristics:
• skin temperature (warmth or coolness)

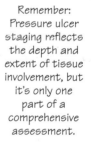

Remember: Pressure ulcer staging reflects the depth and extent of tissue involvement, but it's only one part of a comprehensive assessment.

- tissue consistency (boggy or firm)
- sensation (pain or itching).

This ulcer presents clinically as a defined area of persistent redness in patients with light skin or persistent red, blue, or purple in patients with darker skin.

Stage II

A stage II pressure ulcer is a superficial partial-thickness wound that presents clinically as an abrasion, a blister, or a shallow crater involving the epidermis and dermis.

Stage III

A stage III pressure ulcer is a full-thickness wound with tissue damage or necrosis of subcutaneous tissue that can extend down to, but not through, underlying fasciae. The ulcer presents clinically as a deep crater with or without undermining of adjacent tissue.

Stage IV

A stage IV ulcer involves full-thickness skin loss with extensive damage, destruction, or necrosis to muscle, bone, and supporting structures (such as tendons and joint capsule). Undermining and sinus tracts may be present as well.

Closed pressure ulcers

Although the pathology is the same, closed pressure ulcers are unique and potentially life-threatening pressure ulcers. They begin when shearing force causes ischemic necrosis in subcutaneous tissue. No surface defect marks this event. In time, pressure from inflammation in the cavity of necrotic debris causes a small, unremarkable ulcer to form on the skin. This ulcer drains a large contaminated base. There are no signs of systemic infection either.

A class of their own

Closed pressure ulcers can't be classified by stage or grade because it's impossible to determine the extent of damage until the defect is surgically opened. In addition, surgery is the only viable treatment.

Patients confined to wheelchairs because of spinal cord injury are at highest risk for this type of pressure ulcer, and the ulcers occur most commonly in the pelvic region. Prompt recognition is crucial. The only viable treatment is wide surgical excision and closure with a muscle rotation flap.

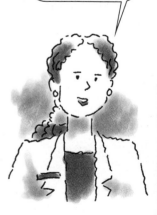

Patients who are confined to wheelchairs are at greatest risk for closed pressure ulcers.

Treatment

Treatment of pressure ulcers follows the four basic steps common to all wound care:

Debride necrotic tissue and clean the wound to remove debris.

Provide a moist wound-healing environment through the use of proper dressings.

Protect the wound from further injury.

Provide nutrition essential to wound healing.

A key element in all pressure ulcer treatment plans is identifying and treating, when possible, the underlying pathophysiology. If the cause of the ulcer remains, existing ulcers don't heal and new ulcers develop.

Typically, wound care involves cleaning the wound, debriding necrotic tissue, and applying a dressing that keeps the wound bed moist. Topical agents are used to resolve various issues.

Wound cleaning

Wound cleaning removes wound debris, old dressing materials, and necrotic tissue from the wound surface. Pressurized wound irrigation is adequate for almost all wound cleaning. (For more information on wound cleaning, see chapter 3, Basic wound care procedures.)

Debridement

Debridement removes nonviable tissue and is the most important factor in wound management. Healing can't take place until necrotic tissue is removed. (For more information on debridement, see chapter 3, Basic wound care procedures.)

Dressings

Dressings serve to:
- protect the wound from contamination
- prevent trauma
- provide compression (if bleeding or swelling occurs)
- apply medications
- absorb drainage or debride necrotic tissue.

When choosing a dressing for a pressure ulcer, the cardinal rule remains the same: Keep moist tissue moist and dry tissue dry. Wound characteristics dictate the type of dressing used. The dressing selected should protect wound integrity and keep the wound surface moist but prevent an excessive buildup of moisture, which can cause maceration and bacterial colonization. The frequency of dressing changes depends on the amount and type of wound drainage as well as the characteristics of the dressing.

Wound cavities may require light packing or fill to prevent areas from walling off and developing into abscesses. Be careful with packing though; too much packing can generate more pressure and cause additional tissue damage.

Patient education

Remember that the goal of patient education is to improve the outcome. For any care plan to succeed after the patient leaves the hospital, the patient or caregiver must understand the care plan, be physically capable of carrying it out at home, and value both the information and the outcomes. Therefore, education and goal establishment should take into consideration the preferences and lifestyles of the patient and his family whenever possible.

Teach the patient and family members how to prevent pressure ulcers and what to do when they occur. (See *Pressure ulcer do's*

Get wise to wounds

Pressure ulcer do's and don'ts

With proper skin care and frequent position changes, patients and their caregivers can keep the patient's skin healthy—a crucial element in pressure ulcer prevention. Here are some important do's and don'ts to pass along to patients:

Do...
• Change position at least once every 2 hours while reclining. Follow a schedule. Lie on your right side, then your left side, then your back, then your stomach (if possible). Use pillows and pads for support. Make small turns between the 2-hour changes.
• Check your skin for signs of pressure ulcers twice daily. Use a mirror to check areas you can't inspect directly, such as the shoulders, tailbone, hips, elbows, heels, and the back of the head. Report any breaks in the skin or changes in skin temperature to your doctor.

• Follow the prescribed exercise program, including range-of-motion exercises every 8 hours, or as recommended.
• Eat a well-balanced diet, drink lots of fluids, and strive to maintain the recommended weight.

Don't...
• Use commercial soaps or skin products that dry or irritate your skin—use oil-free lotions.
• Sleep on wrinkled bed sheets or tuck your covers tightly into the foot of your bed.

and don'ts.) Explain repositioning, and show them what a 30-degree laterally inclined position looks like. If the patient needs assistance with repositioning, make sure he knows the types of devices available and where he obtain them.

Mirror, mirror...

Show the patient how he can inspect his back and other areas using a mirror. If the patient can't do this, a family member can help. Make sure he understands the importance of inspecting skin over bony prominences for pressure related damage every day.

If the patient needs to apply dressings at home, make sure he knows the proper ways to apply and remove them. Tell him where he can get supplies if he runs low.

Ensuring proper nutrition can be difficult, but the patient and his family need to know how important proper nutrition is to the healing process. Provide materials on nutrition and maintaining an ideal weight, as appropriate. Show them how to create an easy-to-read chart of care reminders for a wall at home.

Pressure ulcers should be reassessed weekly. Measure progress by the reduction in necrotic tissue and drainage and the increase in granulation tissue and epithelial growth. Clean, vascularized pressure ulcers should show evidence of healing within 2 weeks. If they don't and the patient has followed the guidelines for nutrition, repositioning, use of support surfaces, and wound care, it's time to reevaluate the care plan.

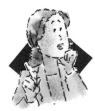

Quick quiz

1. Pressure ulcers are categorized as:
    A.   acute wounds.
    B.   chronic wounds.
    C.   partial-thickness wounds.
    D.   full-thickness wounds.

Answer: B. Pressure ulcers are chronic wounds.

2.   A good way to assess your patient's pressure ulcer risk is to use:
    A.   a review of body systems approach.
    B.   the Kransky Pressure Sore Assessment tool.
    C.   your experience with other pressure ulcer patients.
    D.   the Braden Pressure Sore Risk Assessment Scale.

Answer: D. The Braden Pressure Sore Risk Assessment Scale is used extensively to assess pressure ulcer risk.

3.   Which of the following interventions is most appropriate for preventing excessive heel pressure?

  A.   Flexing the knees.
  B.   Placing a donut-shaped cushion under the feet.
  C.   Suspending the heels by placing a pillow under the calves.
  D.   Putting a pressure reducing foam mattress under the heels.

Answer: C. Suspending the heels using a pillow under the calves is the best way to protect heels from pressure ulceration.

4.   Which body position simultaneously relieves pressure from the sacrum and trochanter?

  A.   Prone
  B.   Supine
  C.   30-degree lateral position
  D.   90-degree side-lying position

Answer: C. A 30-degree lateral position is the best way to relieve pressure from both the sacrum and the trochanter.

5.   A pressure ulcer that appears innocent on the skin surface, but that conceals a deep, walled-off cavity filled with necrotic debris is a:

  A.   closed pressure ulcer.
  B.   stage II pressure ulcer.
  C.   stage III pressure ulcer.
  D.   stage IV pressure ulcer.

Answer: A. A closed pressure ulcer is a deep and potentially fatal lesion.

Scoring

☆☆☆ If you answered all five questions correctly, congratulations! You've certainly demonstrated that you can handle the pressure.

☆☆ If you answered three or four questions correctly, nicely done! You're near the top of the pressure gradient.

☆ If you answered fewer than three questions correctly, don't despair. You'll reposition yourself soon.

Diabetic foot ulcers

Just the facts

In this chapter, you'll learn:

♦ causes of diabetic foot ulcers

♦ assessment criteria for diabetic foot ulcers

♦ interventions for diabetic foot ulcer treatment

♦ prevention measures for diabetic foot ulcers.

A look at diabetic foot ulcers

Diabetes mellitus is a metabolic disorder characterized by hyperglycemia resulting from lack of insulin, lack of insulin effect, or both. Insulin transports glucose into cells, where it's used as fuel or stored as glycogen. Insulin also stimulates protein synthesis and storage of free fatty acids in fat deposits. An insulin deficiency compromises these important functions. Diabetes can begin suddenly or develop insidiously. (See *Diabetes: The not-so-sweet facts.*)

High plasma glucose levels caused by diabetes can damage blood vessels and nerves. Therefore, patients with diabetes are prone to developing foot ulcers due to nerve damage and poor circulation to the lower extremities. Good diabetes control may help prevent these potentially chronic problems or make them less serious.

Causes

Diabetic neuropathy, pressure and other mechanical forces, and poor circulation can cause foot ulcers in patients with diabetes.

Diabetes: The not-so-sweet facts

Diabetes has been characterized as a modern day epidemic, and it isn't hard to understand why when you look at the statistics for the United States:

• Approximately 16 million people—6% of the population—have diabetes.

• Each year, doctors diagnose 798,000 new cases of diabetes.

• Diabetes is the seventh leading cause of death.

• 15% of all persons with diabetes develop diabetic foot ulcers sometime during their life.

• 14% to 20% of patients with diabetic ulcers require amputation.

• Diabetes is most prevalent in African Americans, Hispanics, and Native Americans, and the risk is highest for middle-aged and older adults.

Diabetic neuropathy

Peripheral neuropathy is the primary cause of diabetic foot ulcer development. Neuropathy is a nerve disorder that results in impaired or lost function in the tissues served by the affected nerve fibers. In diabetes, neuropathy may be caused by ischemia due to thickening in the tiny blood vessels that supply the nerve or by nerve demyelinization (destruction of the protective myelin sheath surrounding a nerve), which slows the conduction of impulses.

Polyneuropathy, or damage to multiple types of nerves, is the most common form of neuropathy in patients with diabetes. In the foot, a trineuropathy develops that includes:
- loss of sensation
- loss of motor function
- loss of autonomic functions (the autonomic nervous system controls smooth muscles, glands, and visceral organs). (See *Understanding diabetic trineuropathy*.)

Typically, impairment affects the feet and hands first and then progresses toward the knees and elbows, respectively. This presentation is called a *stocking and glove distribution.*

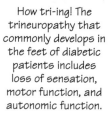

Feeling impulsive? Nerve obstruction or destruction can slow impulse conduction, leading to diabetic foot ulcer development.

You've lost that warning feeling

As sensory nerves degenerate and die (sensory neuropathy), the patient experiences a burning or "pins-and-needles" sensation that might worsen at night.

As sensation declines, the patient risks foot injury. Impaired sensation prevents the patient from feeling stimuli, such as pain and pressure, that normally warn of impending damage. Anything from stepping on something sharp to wearing ill-fitting shoes can result in foot injury because the patient can't feel the damage happening.

A-trophy that isn't a prize

As motor nerves degenerate and die (motor neuropathy), muscles in the limbs atrophy, especially the intrinsic muscles of the feet, which causes footdrop and structural deformities. These degenerative changes increase the patient's risk of stumbling or falling and further damaging the foot.

There's a bad infection on the rise

As autonomic nerves degenerate and die (autonomic neuropathy), sweat and sebaceous glands malfunction and skin on the patient's feet dries and cracks. If fissures develop, the risk of infection rises.

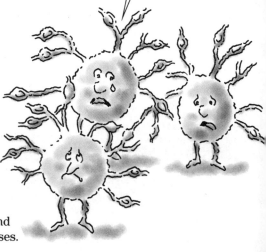

How tri-ing! The trineuropathy that commonly develops in the feet of diabetic patients includes loss of sensation, motor function, and autonomic function.

Now I get it!

Understanding diabetic trineuropathy

Uncontrolled diabetes commonly results in a trineuropathy (three concurrent neuropathies) that dramatically increases the patient's risk of developing diabetic foot ulcers.

Sensory neuropathy

In sensory neuropathy, ischemia or demyelinization (see illustration below) causes nerve death or deterioration. When this occurs, the patient no longer feels painful stimuli and, therefore, can no longer respond appropriately.

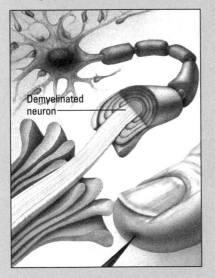

Demyelinated neuron

Motor neuropathy

In motor neuropathy, intrinsic muscles deep in the plantar surface of the foot atrophy, resulting in increased arch height and clawed toes. In addition, the fat pad that normally covers the metatarsal heads migrates toward the toes, exposing the metatarsal heads to more pressure and increasing pressure ulcer

risk. The risk is high for the upper surfaces of claw toes as well, especially if the patient has poorly fitted shoes.

The illustration below shows the degenerative changes in the foot resulting from motor neuropathy. Shading indicates the areas where ulcers are most likely to develop.

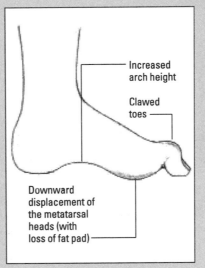

Increased arch height

Clawed toes

Downward displacement of the metatarsal heads (with loss of fat pad)

Autonomic neuropathy

In uncontrolled diabetes, autonomic neuropathy inhibits or destroys the sympathetic component of the autonomic nervous system, which controls vasoconstriction in peripheral blood vessels. The resulting unfettered flow of blood to the lower limbs and feet may cause os-

teopenia (reduction of bone volume) in foot and ankle bones.

In Charcot disease (neuropathic osteoarthropathy), the bones weakened by osteopenia suffer fractures that the patient doesn't feel due to sensory neuropathy. Over time, this process causes bony dissolution that culminates with the collapse of the midfoot into a rocker bottom deformity (see illustration below). Patients with Charcot disease are placed on non-weight-bearing status until inflammation subsides.

Midfoot ulcers resulting from increased plantar pressures over the rocker bottom deformity heal slower than ulcers on the forefoot.

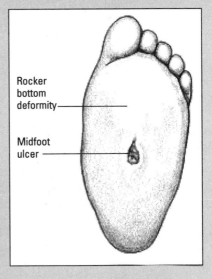

Rocker bottom deformity

Midfoot ulcer

Mechanical forces

Mechanical forces involved in diabetic ulcer generation include pressure, friction, and shear.

Pressure

Sensory neuropathy places a patient at increased risk for diabetic foot ulcers caused by pressure — especially a patient who's confined to a bed or wheelchair. Such a patient can suffer damage simply by letting his feet rest for too long on a bed or a wheelchair footrest. Impaired sensation prevents the patient from feeling the discomfort that results from staying in one position too long.

Prominent plantar pressure places

As with pressure ulcers, areas over bony prominences are the most common places for diabetic foot ulcers, including:
- the metatarsal heads
- the great toe
- the heel.

Friction and shear

Although pressure is the major mechanical force at work in the development of diabetic ulcers, it isn't the only one. Friction and shear can cause damage as well. A loose shoe rubbing against the foot or a foot sliding across a bed sheet can cause friction damage.

Shearly it's no jest

Shearing forces build up when damp skin sticks to a surface while the underlying bone and tissue move. For example, the skin of a sweating foot can cling to a shoe while the underlying tissues slide beneath the skin.

Peripheral vascular disease

Peripheral vascular disease (PVD), a common problem in patients with diabetes, impairs the healing process of existing ulcers and may contribute to neuropathy as well. In PVD, atherosclerosis narrows the peripheral arteries, slowly reducing the flow of blood to the limbs. (See *How atherosclerosis impairs circulation*.) As perfusion drops, the risks of ischemia and tissue necrosis increase.

Now I get it!

How atherosclerosis impairs circulation

In atherosclerosis, fatty deposits (cholesterol) and fibrous plaques accumulate along the walls of the arteries, narrowing the lumen and reducing the artery's elasticity. Thrombi (blood clots) form on the roughened surface of plaques and may grow large enough to block the artery's lumen.

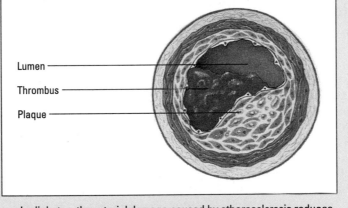

Lumen

Thrombus

Plaque

In diabetes, the arterial damage caused by atherosclerosis reduces blood flow to the lower limbs and to the nerves that innervate them. In addition to promoting ulcer development, poor perfusion slows the healing process for existing ulcers and impedes circulation of systemic antibiotics to infected areas.

Assessment

Assessment of diabetic foot ulcers includes a thorough patient history, a physical examination, and special testing of the lower extremities.

History

A thorough patient history is key to assessing diabetic foot ulcers. In addition to the basic information elicited during a traditional patient history, ask the patient about:
• date of onset of diabetes

- management measures
- medications
- other diagnosed problems
- status and history of any diagnosed neuropathy
- allergies, especially skin reactions
- tobacco and alcohol use
- recent changes in activity level
- date and location of previous ulcerations
- date that he first noticed the current ulcer
- the way in which the ulcer occurred
- type and quality of any associated pain.

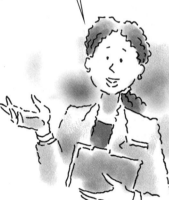

Treat the body as a unit, and remember, a thorough assessment of the patient's condition requires examination of several systems.

Physical examination

Use a holistic approach when performing the physical examination. Remember that the patient's overall physical health and state of mind affect wound healing.

The general physical examination evaluates the patient's musculoskeletal, neurologic, vascular, and integumentary systems to provide perspective for assessing the condition of the lower limbs.

Boning up

Assess these aspects of the patient's musculoskeletal system:
- posture
- gait
- strength, flexibility, and endurance
- range of motion.

Making connections

Assess these aspects of the patient's neurologic system:
- balance
- reflexes
- sensory function.

Flowing smoothly

Assess these aspects of the patient's vascular system:
- posterior tibial and dorsalis pedis pulses
- ankle-brachial index (ABI).

Getting the skinny

Assess these aspects of the patient's integumentary system:
- texture
- temperature
- color
- appendages (hair, sweat glands, sebaceous glands, nails).

Features of diabetic foot ulcers

In diabetic foot ulcers, characteristic clinical features depend on the location of the ulcer.

Ulcer location	Clinical features
Plantar surface	Even wound margins
Great toe	Deep wound bed
Metatarsal head	Dry or low to moderate exudate
Heel	Low to moderate exudate
Tip or top of toe	Pale granulation with ischemia or bright-red, friable granulation tissue with infection

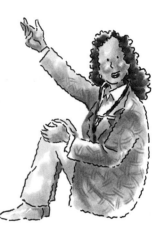

Foot examination

An evaluation of the patient's feet is central to detecting and assessing diabetic foot ulcers. Check the following high-risk areas of the feet for existing or impending ulcers (calluses, for example):
• plantar surfaces (soles) of the toes
• tips of the toes
• between the toes
• lateral aspect of the foot's plantar surface.

Wound characteristics depend on where the wound occurs on the foot. (See *Features of diabetic foot ulcers*.) Characteristics of surrounding skin may include:
• calluses (considered prewounds)
• blood blisters (hemorrhage beneath a callus)
• erythema, indicating inflammation or infection
• induration (hardened edges)
• skin fissures (portals for bacterial entry)
• dry, scaly skin.

Special testing

Special tests provide a clearer picture of the health of the lower leg and foot. These tests evaluate pressure, neurologic function, and perfusion. The results provide insight into the mechanism of injury, condition of the wound bed and surrounding tissue, prognosis for healing, and required treatment interventions.

Musculoskeletal tests

Harris mat prints and computerized pressure mapping are special musculoskeletal tests that provide information about the plantar pressures of the foot.

Harris mat prints

Pressure over bony prominences is one cause of diabetic foot ulcers. A simple method for determining areas of increased pressure on the plantar surface of the foot is to use an ink mat.

Making an impression

In Harris mat prints, the examiner inks the bottom of the mat, which has a grid to aid assessment of results, and places it on an evaluation template or clean sheet of paper. Then the patient steps on the uninked top surface of the mat, placing equal weight on each foot. If needed, the examiner holds the patient's outstretched hands to help ensure equal weight distribution. The impression on the template or sheet of paper shows relative areas of pressure under the patient's foot. Darker areas on the grid indicate high-pressure areas. In a case where a dynamic impression is required, the patient slowly walks across the mat to create the impression.

> I can't predict everything. In Harris mat prints and computerized pressure mapping, footprints can foretell possible problem regions by identifying areas of high pressure.

Under pressure

High-pressure areas usually correlate with calluses (prewounds) or existing wounds. The results help guide the choice of special off-loading devices, which help relieve pressure when the patient stands or walks.

Computerized pressure mapping

Computerized pressure mapping devices test plantar pressures while the patient is wearing a shoe and when he's barefoot. The approach is similar to Harris mat prints; however, in this test, a computer maps the pressures and displays the results on a printout. A color gradient illustrates relative pressure, with red and orange indicating areas where pressure is highest.

Neurologic tests

Neurologic tests for the lower extremities include deep tendon reflexes testing, vibration perception testing with a tuning fork or biothesiometer, and Semmes-Weinstein monofilament testing for protective sensation.

Deep tendon reflexes testing

Peripheral neuropathy causes a decrease in deep tendon reflexes. Decreased deep tendon reflexes correlate with muscular atrophy, usually the intrinsic muscles of the foot in a patient with diabetes.

Tuning fork test

In this test, the examiner uses a tuning fork to assess peripheral nerve function and help identify and quantify any neuropathy. Here's how:

Name that tune

- The examiner activates the tuning fork and holds it against a bony prominence in the affected limb—for example, a metatarsal head or malleoli—and then records the patient's ability to sense the vibration.
- Next, the examiner tests other bony prominences in the body, for example the patella or elbow, or the same prominence in the opposite limb if it's unaffected.
- Afterward, the results are compared to assess neurologic function.

Biothesiometer

A biothesiometer is another tool that's used to assess vibratory perception threshhold. It provides a better quantitative measurement of vibratory sense than the tuning fork. Individuals with sensory neuropathy have impaired vibratory perception thresholds (less than 25 volts, as measured on the biothesiometer).

Semmes-Weinstein test

The Semmes-Weinstein test helps determine the level of protective sensation in the feet. While the patient's eyes are closed, the examiner holds the Semmes-Weinstein monofilament perpendicular to the patient's foot and then presses the monofilament against the skin until it bows. The patient is then asked to identify when and where the skin has been touched. As protective sensation decreases, plantar pressures tend to rise, as does the patient's risk of ulcers at these points. (See *Performing the Semmes-Weinstein test*, page 164.)

Vascular tests

Vascular tests help assess circulation in the lower extremities. These tests include pulse palpation, ABI, toe pressures, and transcutaneous oxygen ($TcPO_2$) levels.

Pulse palpation

Initial assessment of limb perfusion includes palpating the dorsalis pedis, posterior tibial, popliteal, and femoral pulses. If it's hard to

Performing the Semmes-Weinstein test

The Semmes-Weinstein test uses a special monofilament to help assess protective sensation in the patient's feet. The illustration below shows the points to test, which include:
- plantar surface of the first, third, and fifth toes
- first, third, and fifth metatarsal heads
- lateral and medial midfoot
- midheel
- middorsal surface of the foot.

How it's done
The examiner places the 10 g monofilament on one of the testing points and exerts enough pressure to bow the monofilament, as illustrated below. With his eyes closed, the patient must then identify where and when he's touched.

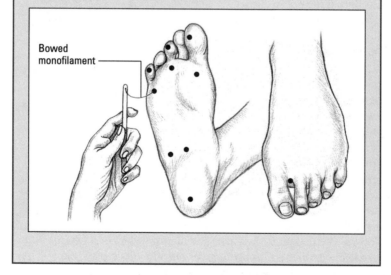

Bowed monofilament

palpate a pulse due to edema, consider using Doppler ultrasound, which produces an audible signal coinciding with the pulse.

Feel the beat

Hold the transducer at a 45-degree angle to the skin and listen for the beats. The results provide a general idea of the circulation to each level of the limb. A palpable dorsalis pedis pulse is roughly equiva-

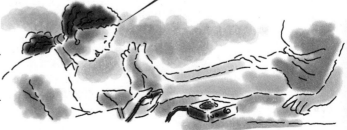

Listen up! If edema makes the patient's pulse hard to palpate, you may want to use Doppler ultrasound.

Rate that pulse!

When assessing the amplitude of a pulse, rate the strength on a numerical scale or use a specific descriptive term. You can use the scale below to rate that pulse!

Rating	Pulse characteristic
0	No palpable pulse
+1	Weak or thready pulse: hard to feel, easily obliterated by slight finger pressure
+2	Normal pulse: easily palpable, obliterated by strong finger pressure
+3	Bounding pulse: readily palpable, forceful, not easily obliterated by finger pressure

---

lent to 80 mm Hg, which is adequate for healing most diabetic wounds. (See *Rate that pulse!*)

Ankle-brachial index

PVD and resulting poor perfusion are common problems for patients with diabetes. Poor perfusion increases the patient's likelihood of developing ulcers and reduces the speed with which existing ulcers heal—a double whammy. ABI is used in conjunction with other vascular tests to determine and monitor the patient's risk of ischemia in the area of the ankle. ABI is a ratio of systolic blood pressure in the brachial artery in the arm to systolic blood pressure measured in the dorsalis pedis artery in the ankle. (For more information on ABI, see chapter 6, Pressure ulcers.)

Toe pressures

Toe pressures may be a more sensitive indicator of changes in vascular integrity in the distal areas of the foot. Toe pressures are performed in the same manner as limb blood pressures, except that a much smaller, specialized cuff is used for the toe. Due to the tiny arteries in digits, the corresponding arterial pressures are lower than those measured in an arm or leg. Typical pressure in the toe is about 70% of systolic values obtained in the arm.

What toe pressure tells you

Toe pressures allow you to gauge the patient's ischemic risk profile. Generally, toe pressure:
- above 55 mm Hg reflects a low risk of tissue ischemia.
- below 40 mm Hg reflects a high risk of ischemia.

- below 20 mm Hg reflects a severe risk of ischemia.
- of 45 mm Hg or higher is needed for healing to occur.

Transcutaneous oxygen level

$TcPO_2$ levels reflect the oxygen saturation of tissues. Typically, $TcPO_2$ levels are measured close to the ulcer. In general, a $TcPO_2$ level:

- above 40% reflects a low risk of tissue ischemia
- between 20% and 30% reflects a high risk of ischemia
- below 20% reflects a severe risk of ischemia
- of 30% or higher is required for healing.

Classification

Diabetic foot ulcers are classified according to depth, presence of ischemia, and presence of infection, depending on the classification system. The Wagner Ulcer Grade Classification System and the University of Texas Wound Classification System for Diabetic Foot Ulcers are two commonly used classification systems.

Wagner Ulcer Grade

In the Wagner Ulcer Grade Classification System, less complex ulcers receive lower scores; more complex ulcers, higher scores. Ulcers with higher scores may require surgical intervention or amputation.

Grade	Characteristics
0	• Preulcer lesion • Healed ulcer • Presence of bony deformity
1	• Superficial ulcer without subcutaneous tissue involvement
2	• Penetration through the subcutaneous tissue; may expose bone, tendon, ligament, or joint capsule
3	• Osteitis, abscess, or osteomyelitis
4	• Gangrene of a digit
5	• Gangrene requiring foot amputation

Adapted with permission from Glugla, M., and Mulder, G.D., "The Diabetic Foot: Medical Management of Foot Ulcers," in *Chronic Wound Care*. Edited by Krasner, D. King of Prussia, Pa.: Health Management Publications, Inc., 1990.

University of Texas classification system

The University of Texas Wound Classification System for Diabetic Foot Ulcers provides a detailed categorization of diabetic foot ulcers. This system allows for the consideration of infection and ischemia.

Stage	Grade 0	Grade I	Grade II	Grade III
A	Preulcerative or postulcerative foot at risk for further ulceration	Superficial ulcer without tendon, capsule, or bone involvement	Ulcer penetrating to tendon or joint capsule	Ulcer penetrating to bone
B	Presence of infection	Presence of infection	Presence of infection	Presence of infection
C	Presence of ischemia	Presence of ischemia	Presence of ischemia	Presence of ischemia
D	Presence of infection and ischemia	Presence of infection and ischemia	Presence of infection and ischemia	Presence of infection and ischemia

Adapted with permission from "Best Practices for the Prevention, Diagnosis, and Treatment of Diabetic Foot Ulcers," *Ostomy/Wound Management* 46(11):55-68, November 2000.

Wagner Ulcer Grade Classification System

The original Wagner Ulcer Grade Classification System considers depth of penetration; however, it doesn't allow for the assessment of infection at all tissue levels. A modified version of the Wagner classification system adds levels to take into account infection and ischemia. (See *Wagner Ulcer Grade.*)

University of Texas Wound Classification System

The University of Texas Wound Classification System for Diabetic Foot Ulcers takes tissue infection and ischemia into consideration and provides a more detailed breakdown of classifications than the Wagner system. (See *University of Texas classification system.*)

Complications

The most common complications that impede the healing of diabetic foot ulcers include:

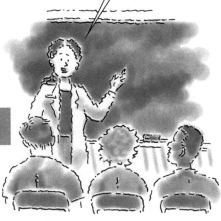

At the head of the class are the Wagner Ulcer Grade and University of Texas classification systems for diabetic foot ulcers.

• multiple comorbidities, including PVD—cause a number of problems that increase the risk of ulceration and reduce the likelihood of speedy healing

• uncontrolled hyperglycemia—commonly signals infection and inhibits the immune system, particularly the scavenging function of neutrophils

• psychosocial problems, such as depression and poverty—profoundly affect the patient's nutritional status, which in turn affects the body's ability to prevent ulcers and heal existing wounds.

Any of these complications can cause a wound to become chronic.

> Comorbidities are speed bumps on the remedial road. They can slow healing of existing ulcers and contribute to new ones.

Infection

Infection is a common complication in diabetic foot ulcers. An infection in the wound or elsewhere consumes protein needed for healing and interferes directly by damaging the wound bed.

Scanning for signs

Uncontrollable blood glucose or hyperglycemia may be the first sign of infection because patients with diabetes commonly fail to demonstrate the typical systemic responses. A 4° to 5° difference in temperature between similar areas on each foot is a local sign of infection. An infrared scanner thermometer is the most reliable way to check this difference. An infection in the wound bed commonly causes friable (easy to bleed), bright-red granulation tissue.

Osteomy-oh-my-elitis

Osteomyelitis or bone infection is common in deep wounds. A quick and reliable method for determining whether osteomyelitis is present in a diabetic ulcer bed is to palpate for bone. A palpable bone usually indicates osteomyelitis. However, osteomyelitis may be difficult to distinguish from acute Charcot neuropathic osteoarthropathy. The best way to differentiate between the two is to culture a bone fragment from the wound bed.

> There's no if, ands, or bones about it! If you palpate bone in a diabetic ulcer bed, your patient probably has osteomyelitis. Culture a bone fragment to make sure.

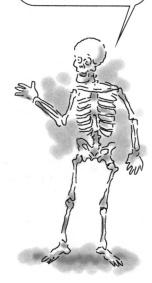

Infection inspection

Infections fall into two categories: limb threatening or non-limb-threatening. Non-limb-threatening infections tend to be superficial infections involving tissues within 2 cm of the wound margin. In this type of infection, no significant tissue ischemia is present and bone isn't palpable in the wound bed. Non-limb-threatening infection can be treated with topical antimicrobials, sharp debridement, and wound cleaning once or twice daily.

In contrast, limb-threatening infection involves tissue more than 2 cm from the wound margin, palpable bone in the wound bed, and tissue ischemia. Hospitalization and surgical debridement of infected bone and soft tissues is requisite. Unless the infected bone is fully resected, the patient requires 4 to 8 weeks of I.V. antibiotic therapy.

Diabetic foot ulcer care

Successful healing depends on proper wound cleaning and dressing and off-loading. Topical antimicrobials, debridement, biotherapies, and surgery may also be included in the care plan.

> Obliterating bacteria is a benefit. Such devices as bulb syringes and syringes with angiocatheters can help make cleaning the wound bed easier.

Wound cleaning

Wound cleaning is a fundamental step in the healing process. Necrotic tissue is a reservoir for bacteria and inhibits wound healing.

Flushing the wound bed with normal saline solution is the best method of cleaning a diabetic foot ulcer. Most commercial wound cleaners are somewhat toxic to cells in the wound bed, and their use can slow healing. Use clean, warm water and mild soap to clean the surrounding skin.

Healing hands

Cleaning the wound bed can be made easier by using bulb syringes, syringes with angiocatheters, aerosolized saline in a canister, pulsatile lavage with suction, and whirlpool. (For more information on wound cleaning, see chapter 3, Basic wound care procedures.)

Wound dressings

Moist wound therapy speeds healing in diabetic foot ulcers. Dressings that maintain the necessary wound environment include:
- alginates
- transparent films
- foams
- hydrocolloids
- hydrogels
- collagen-based dressings
- composites (combinations of the other dressings).

Choose wisely

Choice of dressing depends on the condition of the ulcer. Diabetic foot ulcers tend to produce low to moderate drainage. However, if the wound bed is dry, it needs a dressing that adds moisture. Either amorphous hydrogels or sheet hydrogels can help in this case. Hydrogel sheets are more cost-effective but don't work as well in deeper wounds. For deep or tunneling ulcers that require packing, hydrogel impregnated gauze is an excellent alternative to amorphous hydrogels and it costs less. All hydrogel dressings add moisture to the wound bed—they're as much as 95% water themselves. Hydrogels also encourage autolytic debridement. (See *Dressings for diabetic foot ulcers.*)

Relieving pressure from plantar surfaces, which is also known as off-loading, is key to pressure ulcer treatment and prevention.

Off-loading

Off-loading—relieving pressure from—plantar tissues is the cornerstone of diabetic neuropathy treatment as well as prevention for those patients at risk for recurrent breakdown. Off-loading seeks to control, limit, or remove all intrinsic and extrinsic factors that increase plantar pressures. Examples of intrinsic risk factors include faulty biomechanics in the foot or the presence of a bony deformity. Extrinsic risk factors include trauma, ill-fitting shoes, or maintaining a position for too long, allowing the damaging effects of pressure to build up—for example, lying supine in bed or resting a heel against the footrest of a wheelchair.

Step off!

Off-loading is particularly important because patients with diabetic neuropathy can no longer feel the growing discomfort that precedes tissue damage. Off-loading pressure prevents or limits the kind of tissue damage that causes ulcers to form.

Nonsurgical off-loading techniques

Off-loading can be accomplished using nonsurgical or surgical interventions. Nonsurgical interventions include therapeutic footwear, possibly with rocker soles; custom orthotics; and walking casts. When considering a device for a patient, keep in mind that using a device can increase the patient's risk of falling. If this is true for your patient, be sure to provide instruction on fall prevention.

Dress for success

Dressings for diabetic foot ulcers

Use the chart below to help you choose an appropriate dressing for your patient's foot ulcer.

Type of ulcer	Recommended dressings
Dry ulcer	• Hydrogel
Wet ulcer	• Alginate • Foam • Collagen
Necrotic ulcer	• Hydrogel • Hydrocolloid
Shallow ulcer	• Transparent film • Hydrocolloid
Tunneling or deep ulcer	• Alginate ropes (for wet ulcers) • Hydrogel impregnated gauze (for dry ulcers)
Infected ulcer	• Iodosorb (a gel that cleans the wound by absorbing fluid, exudate, and bacteria) • Acticoat or Arglaes (products with an antimicrobial component)
Bleeding ulcer	• Alginate

Shoes

Good shoes are important. For a patient with no loss of protective sensation, this may equate to a comfortable, well-fitting pair of tennis shoes. At the other end of the spectrum, a patient with recurring ulcers and severe foot deformities needs a custom-molded shoe. Common design features of therapeutic footwear include:
• soft, breathable leather that conforms to foot deformities
• high tops for ankle stability
• rocker soles and bottoms for pressure and pain relief across the plantar metatarsal heads
• a toe box with extra-depth and width to accommodate deformities, such as claw toes and hallux valgus (displacement of the great toe toward the other toes)
• flared lateral soles for stability. (See *Therapeutic shoe modifications*, page 172.)

Therapeutic shoe modifications

These illustrations show the modifications in custom shoes that can improve stability and accommodate the deformities that affect many patients with diabetes.

High top

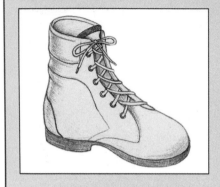

Lateral flare

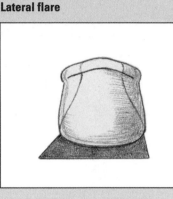

Rocker sole

Custom orthotics

Custom orthotics are shoe inserts that serve various functions based on the patient's needs. In general, custom orthotics relieve pressure, reduce shearing force and friction, and cushion the foot against shocks. If necessary, custom orthotics accommodate the patient's foot deformities as well.

Walking casts

Walking casts range from total contact casts to splints and walkers.

Cast member

A total contact cast is the top of the line in care for uninfected diabetic ulcers on the plantar surface of the foot. Total contact casts are custom made for each patient by a health care professional, typically a physical therapist or orthotist. Inside the cast, padding is fitted over bony areas of the ankle and leg that are at risk for pressure ulcers. A plaster shell reinforced with plaster splints covers the padding. Fiberglass covers the plaster to lend rigidity and additional strength. The cast includes a sturdy walking heel for ambulation. The cast is molded to fit snugly to prevent the foot from sliding inside the cast. This reduces shearing forces over the plantar surface.

A patient with an infected diabetic ulcer isn't a candidate for a total contact cast because a cast makes daily assessment, cleaning, and antimicrobial therapy impossible. In addition, inflammation and edema can cause a buildup of pressure within the cast

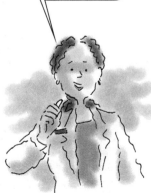

A total contact cast is out of the question for a patient with an infected foot ulcer. Instead, use a removable off-loading device.

and subsequent tissue damage. In the case of infection, a removable off-loading device is the way to go.

Walk this way

Splints and walkers have cushioned inserts with an outer shell of fiberglass or copolymer. Several splint and walker options are available. Splints and walkers have some advantages of their own. For example, they allow easy inspection of the ulcer. In addition, off-loading modifications can be accomplished relatively easy by changing the type of walker or splint in use. However, these devices have disadvantages as well. First and foremost, they don't provide the same degree of pressure and shear relief as a total contact cast. Also, for these therapies to work, the patient must be committed to using the device — a patient can always take a splint off or choose not to use a walker on any given day.

Surgical interventions

Surgical off-loading procedures include surgical dissection of the wound bed and pressure-inducing bony tissue deformities. Pressure over bony prominences compresses and occludes blood vessels, causing ischemia. Resection (surgical removal) of bony deformities reduces peak plantar pressures. This type of surgery is called *curative surgery* because it removes the pathologic tissue. Examples of curative surgery include: exostectomy, digital arthroplasty, bone and joint resections, and partial calcanectomy.

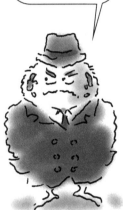

Argh! Foiled again! Using a topical antimicrobial on the wound bed helps keep out microorganisms like me. That improves healing!

Topical antimicrobials

Routine wound cleaning handles much of the surface microbial population. However, applying a topical antimicrobial directly to the wound bed can help control microorganisms in the wound bed and improve healing. Commonly used topical antimicrobials include:
- bacitracin (Baciguent)
- metronidazole (MetroGel)
- mupirocin (Bactroban)
- silver sulfadiazine (Silvadene).

Keep in mind that some microorganisms are resistant to certain topical agents. Also, recent findings indicate that neomycin-containing products, such as Neosporin, can cause allergic reactions. Consequently, these are no longer recommended for ulcer treatment.

The next generation

Newer wound care antimicrobials include: Iodosorb gel, Iodoflex pad, Arglaes antimicrobial barrier, and Acticoat. These products contain iodine or silver, which kills or inhibits microbes. The active ingredients are released slowly in concentrations that are toxic to microbes but not to important cells, such as fibroblasts, in the wound bed. As an added benefit, research seems to indicate that microbes aren't as likely to develop resistance to this new generation of products.

Debridement

Debriding necrotic and nonviable tissue, foreign matter, and microbes from the wound bed expedites wound healing. Surgical debridement, the most effective method of debridement, is required in cases of osteomyelitis or when the wound involves a deep abscess or spreading tissue infection. Sharp debridement, which can be performed at the bedside, is an option when surgery isn't necessary or the patient is a poor surgical candidate. Topical proteolytic enzymes can be applied to wound tissue to augment debridement between sessions. (For more information on wound debridement, see chapter 3, Basic wound care procedures.)

> To provide the best care for your patient, always be aware of the latest and greatest wound care products.

Biotherapies

Growth factors and living skin equivalents are two forms of biotherapy that may be included in the care plan for a patient with a diabetic foot ulcer.

Growth factors

Growth factors orchestrate healing in the wound bed. One factor in particular—platelet-derived growth factor (PDGF)—is called the *master factor*. PDGF plays a central role by stimulating chemotaxis and the proliferation of neutrophils, fibroblasts, and monocytes. In clinical trials, the PDGF-based product, becaplermin (Regranex gel 0.01%), increased wound closure rates. However, this therapy also relies on an adequate vascular supply and proper wound bed preparation.

Living skin equivalents

Living skin equivalents are products composed of living cells and a matrix, or scaffolding, that serves as the extracellular medium. These products act as interactive wound coverings, providing growth factors and other needed molecules. Dermagraft is one example of a living skin equivalent. It has viable fibroblasts that enhance wound healing rates in diabetic ulcers. Graftskin (Apligraf), another living skin equivalent, also accelerates wound healing.

> Living skin equivalents, such as Dermagraft, contribute viable fibroblasts that enhance diabetic ulcer healing.

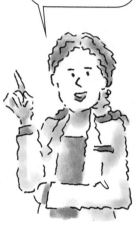

Prevention

Diabetic ulcer prevention starts with identifying the patient's risk factors and then teaching him how to eliminate or minimize these risks.

Identifying risks

Identifying your patient's risk factors is an important part of prevention. Loss of sensation is the single biggest risk factor, but it isn't the only one. Here's a list of risk factors for diabetic ulcers compiled by the American College of Foot and Ankle Surgeons:
* structural foot deformity (such as claw toes, rocker bottom, or hallux vagus)
* trauma and improperly fitted shoes
* calluses
* prior history of ulcerations or amputation
* prolonged, elevated pressure on areas of tissue
* limited joint mobility
* uncontrolled hyperglycemia
* prolonged history of diabetes
* blindness or partial sight
* chronic renal disease
* advanced age.

> Teaching your patient how to eliminate or minimize risk factors is the best form of prevention.

Patient teaching

The next step in prevention is patient education, including teaching about ulcer care and prevention and the importance of controlling diabetes, including the consequences of not controlling it — for example, teaching that poorly controlled blood glucose levels can lead to peripheral neuropathy and vascular damage. Research indicates that tight glycemic control reduces the frequency and severity of neuropathy in individuals with type 1 diabetes. Similar findings have been shown for individuals with type 2 diabetes.

Teach the patient proper foot care and steps he can take to prevent ulcers, including daily examinations, skin washing and maintenance techniques, toenail care, and exercise. Also instruct the patient on how to choose proper socks and shoes. (See *Keeping it toe-gether: Proper foot care,* page 176.)

> **Get wise to wounds**
>
> ## Keeping it toe-gether: Proper foot care
>
> With proper skin care and frequent position changes, patients and their caregivers can keep the patient's skin healthy—a crucial element in pressure ulcer prevention. Here are some important dos and don'ts to pass along to patients.
>
> **Foot care**
> - Check feet daily for injury or pressure areas (a long-handled mirror can help).
> - Wash feet with a mild soap and dry thoroughly between toes.
> - Check bath water to make sure it isn't too hot (test water with your elbow, if able; otherwise, use a thermometer or ask a family member to help).
> - Apply a moisturizing cream (Vaseline is cheap and effective) to prevent dry, cracking skin on the feet and to balance skin pH. Don't apply moisturizer between the toes.
> - Cut toenails off squarely; see a podiatrist if they're dystrophic (deformed and thickened).
> - Don't go barefooted—the risk of injury is too great.
>
> **Socks**
> - Use silver ion-lined socks for fungus control.
> - Wear white or light-colored socks so that bleeding from trauma can be detected quickly.
>
> - Wear natural fiber socks—they breathe better than synthetics.
> - Wear socks that wick perspiration away from feet to prevent maceration.
> - Use diabetic padded socks for shear and friction control.
>
> **Shoes**
> - Wear well-fitting shoes, not shoes that are too tight or loose.
> - Wear shoes that breathe to reduce maceration and fungal infections.
> - With new shoes, wear them for short periods (under 1 hour) each day initially; gradually increase the time as your feet adjust.
> - If deformities are present or you have a history of ulceration, wear professionally fitted shoes.
> - Wash shoes, if possible, to destroy microorganisms.
> - Check shoes before putting them on to make sure nothing fell in that could cause harm.

A clean sock a day keeps the doctor away

White cotton-blended socks are the best choice for a patient with diabetes. Cotton-blended socks wick away moisture and allow air to circulate around the foot. White socks vividly show blood or exudate from an injury or ulcer that the patient may not feel. Regardless of the material, socks should always be nonconstricting and seamless over bony prominences. Socks with added padding can provide additional cushioning as well as some protection from shearing force.

Team effort

Successful prevention programs for diabetic ulcers begin with health promotion. Your patient is at the center of the health care team—all activity focuses on his health needs. In this team, the patient plays an active role in setting personal health care goals, working in partnership with the health care team, who can help him achieve those goals.

Most patients with diabetes have multiple disorders, requiring a series of interventions involving many health disciplines—nurses, doctors, physical therapists, occupational therapists, nutrition-ists, podiatrists, endocrinologists, psychologists, diabetes educa-tors, prosthetists or orthotists, and social workers.

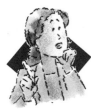

Quick quiz

1. The single greatest risk factor for diabetic foot ulcers is:
  A. PVD.
  B. peripheral neuropathy.
  C. retinitis pigmentosa.
  D. myopathy.

Answer: B. Peripheral neuropathy is the primary risk factor for diabetic foot ulcers.

2. Diabetic ulceration can commonly be found:
  A. around the ankle.
  B. over the sacrum.
  C. on the dorsal surface of the foot.
  D. on the plantar surface of the foot.

Answer: D. Always check the plantar surfaces of the feet for signs of ulcerations. Also check between toes and on the tips of toes.

3. Which of the following complications commonly results from motor neuropathy?
  A. Charcot neuropathic osteoarthropathy
  B. Diminished sensation
  C. Claw toes
  D. Poor circulation

Answer: C. Claw toes commonly result from motor neuropathy, a long-term complication of diabetes.

4. The Semmes-Weinstein test is used to assess:
  A. blood flow to the feet.
  B. protective sensation of the feet.
  C. pressure on the feet.
  D. temperature of the feet.

Answer: B. The Semmes-Weinstein test uses a monofilament to assess the patient's protective sensation, or the ability to detect stimuli that may be harmful to the feet.

5. Which of the following statements is true of the total contact cast?

    A.   It's a method of relieving pressure on the foot.

    B.   It's a special cast for fractures due to Charcot neuropathic osteoarthropathy.

    C.   It's recommended for use over infected diabetic foot ulcerations.

    D.   It's removable.

Answer: A. The total contact cast is an off-loading device that relieves pressure on the foot. However, because it isn't removable, it isn't recommended for use over infected wounds.

Scoring

☆☆☆   If you answered all five questions correctly, you've got a reason to grin! You off-loaded this quiz in a jiffy.

☆☆   If you answered three or four questions correctly, brag to your friends! You zipped through this quiz with no friction, no shear.

☆   If you answered fewer than three questions correctly, let out a sigh, plantar your feet, and move onward and upward!

Wound care products

Just the facts

In this chapter, you'll learn:

♦ types of dressings used in wound care and the characteristics, indications, advantages, and disadvantages of each type

♦ products that are used in conjunction with dressings, including their indications, advantages, and disadvantages

♦ criteria to use when selecting wound care products.

Welcome to the wound care marketplace

The abundance of commercially prepared dressings and adjunct products — and the fact that many have similar names and functions — can make choosing the right product a daunting task.

Over time, wound care has developed from a fairly rudimentary practice that focused primarily on care of the injury to a process that considers the complexities of the patient's general health, possible underlying disease, and specific wound characteristics. As wound care knowledge increased, so did the number and types of products available to aid healing.

In this chapter, we'll look at basic and advanced wound care products and the indications, advantages, and disadvantages of each. As you read, keep in mind that the products discussed here are tools that can help promote full healing, but they aren't the only tools you need. Unless concurrent problems such as malnutrition, circulatory disorders, and patient knowledge deficits are also addressed, the healing process stalls. In addition, no wound care dressing or topical agent can compensate for an incomplete assessment. In short, let the findings of a thorough assessment guide your wound care product selection. (See *Product selection: Let the big picture be your guide*, page 180.)

Product selection: Let the big picture be your guide

When selecting wound care products, let the big picture guide your choices. Ask yourself these important questions:
• Which companies have contracts to supply wound care products to your facility? (Learn about these products first.)
• What's the simplest method of closing the wound? Which is most cost-effective?
• Can the patient afford the supplies he needs? (Simple and affordable aren't necessarily synonymous!) If not, is financial assistance available?
• Who provides wound care at home? If the patient can't perform this important task, can family members or friends? Is home health care an option? If so, is the patient eligible?
• What caused the wound, and how can the cause best be alleviated? (This is especially important when treating chronic wounds; less so when treating acute wounds.)
• How often does the dressing need to be changed? (It takes several hours—figure at least 8 hours—for a wound to achieve homeostasis after a dressing change. Therefore, less often is better!)
• How much drainage is present?
• Does the wound need more moisture?
• Should the wound be debrided? If so, which method is best for the patient?
• After cleaning and drying, does the wound (not the dressing) have an unpleasant odor? Do you suspect infection? If so, is a culture warranted?
• Is there tunneling, undermining, or a cavity that needs to be filled?
• Are the wound edges open or closed? (Wound edges must be open for complete healing to occur.)
• How large is the wound? Would it be more cost-effective to use an advanced wound care product to facilitate granulation tissue or closure?

Keep in touch!

Given the number of products available now, it's hard to believe that there could be anything new around the corner. The truth is that new products arrive almost daily, and others are updated or improved regularly. Because the quality of the care that you provide depends on your level of knowledge, it's imperative that you stay up-to-date by periodically reviewing the products available.

Wound dressings

If we held a wound dressing endurance contest, gauze would win hands-down. Gauze has been a core wound dressing for more years than any other material. However, as medical research has afforded a better understanding of wounds and the healing process, medical manufacturers have developed new materials and sophisticated dressing options that better promote healing.

Moisture level, tissue adherence, infection control, and wound dimensions are just some of the factors that affect wound dressing selection. The level of moisture in the wound bed is critical to the success or failure of healing. Consequently, one fundamental way to classify dressings is by their effect on wound moisture. In other

Dressing for the occasion

Some dressings absorb moisture from a wound bed, whereas others add moisture to it. Use the chart below to quickly determine the category of dressing that's appropriate your patient.

MOISTURE SCALE

Absorb moisture		Neutral (maintain existing moisture level)		Add moisture	
• Alginates • Specialty absorptives • VAC device • Gauze	• Foams • Hydrocolloids • Compression dressings	• Composites • Mini-VAC device	• Transparent films • Biological dressings • Collagen dressings • Contact layers • Warm-Up Therapy System	• Sheet hydrogels	• Amorphous hydrogel • Debriding agents

words, do they add, absorb, or not affect wound moisture? (See *Dressing for the occasion.*)

Gauze but not forgotten

Although gauze remains a good choice for secondary dressings, it no longer represents the most effective choice for a primary dressing. Let's take a close look at the dressings you'll use when providing wound care.

Alginate dressings

Made from seaweed, these nonwoven, absorptive dressings are available as soft, white, sterile pads or ropes. Alginate dressings absorb excessive exudate and may be used on infected wounds. As the dressing absorbs exudate, it turns into a gel that keeps the wound bed moist and promotes healing. Alginates are also nonadhesive and nonocclusive, and they promote autolysis.

Examples of alginate products include:
• AlgiSite M
• KALTOSTAT Wound Dressing
• Maxorb CMC/Alginate Dressing
• Sorbsan Topical Wound Dressing.

Are you looking for a dressing that absorbs moisture? Check out the piece above!

What's the use?

Use alginate dressings on wounds with moderate to heavy drainage.

The good news

Alginate dressings are beneficial because they:
- hold 7 to 10 times their own weight in fluid
- may be cut to fit wound dimensions
- may be layered for more absorption
- come in ropes that are useful for deep wound packing.

The not-so-good news

Irrigation may be needed to remove an alginate dressing from the wound. In addition, alginate dressings:
- require secondary dressings
- can't be used on third-degree burns
- may dehydrate the wound bed of a dryer wound.

Try absorbing this! Alginate dressings are good for wounds with moderate to heavy drainage because they can hold 7 to 10 times their own weight in fluid.

Biological dressings

Biological dressings are temporary dressings that function similarly to skin grafts. They may be made from amnionic or chorionic membranes, woven from manmade fibers, harvested from animals (usually pigs), or harvested from cadavers. These dressings are good only for temporary use because the body eventually rejects them. If rejection occurs before the underlying wound heals, the dressing must be replaced with a skin graft.

Examples of biological dressings include:
- Hyalofill Biopolymeric Wound Dressing
- Inerpan
- Oasis.

What's the use?

Biological dressings should be used as temporary dressings for skin grafting donor sites and burns.

The good news

The biggest advantage of biological dressings is that they can shorten healing times. They also:
- prevent infection and fluid loss
- ease patient discomfort.

The not-so-good news

However, biological dressings:
- are relatively expensive

- may cause allergic reactions
- may require secondary dressings.

Collagen dressings

Collagen dressings, which are made with bovine or avian collagen, accelerate wound healing by encouraging the organization of new collagen fibers and granulation tissue. Examples include:
- FIBRACOL PLUS Collagen Wound Dressing with Alginate
- Kollagen-Medifil Pads.

What's the use?

Collagen dressings should be used on chronic, nonhealing, granulated wound beds.

The good news

Collagen dressings are available in gel, granule, and sheet forms. Some also contain alginate. These dressings are effective on chronic, clean wounds.

The not-so-good news

Disadvantages of collagen dressings include:
- they may cause an allergic reaction if the patient is sensitive to bovine or avian products
- they require secondary dressings
- they aren't appropriate for third-degree burns or on wounds with dry beds.

> Biological dressings may help your patient's wound heal more quickly but beware of allergic reactions.

CAUTION!

Composite dressings

Composite dressings are hybrids that combine two or more types of dressings into one. For example, a three-layer composite dressing can include a bacterial barrier; an absorbent foam, a hydrocolloid, or a hydrogel layer; and an adherent or a nonadherent outer layer. Examples of composite dressings include:
- Alldress
- CompDress Island Dressing
- COVADERM Plus
- MPM Multi-Layered Dressing
- TELFA PLUS Island Dressing.

What's the use?

Composite dressings can be used as the primary or secondary dressings on wounds with light to moderate drainage. They can also be used to protect peripheral and central I.V. lines.

The good news

Composite dressings are:
- all-in-one dressings that come in various combinations, depending on the patient's wound care needs
- available in multiple sizes and shapes.

The not-so-good news

On the other hand, they:
- typically can't manage heavily draining wounds
- can't be cut to fit without losing some of the integrity of the dressing
- can't be used on third-degree burns.

Contact layer dressings

Contact layer dressings are single layers of woven or perforated material suitable for direct contact with the wound's surface. The nonadherent contact layer prevents other dressings from sticking to the surface of the wound. Examples include:
- Conformant 2 Wound Veil
- Mepitel
- Profore Wound Contact Layer
- Telfa Clear.

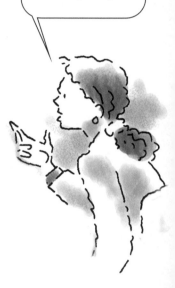

What a relief! Contact layer dressings decrease the pain experienced by the patient during dressing changes.

What's the use?

A contact layer dressing is used to allow the flow of drainage to a secondary dressing while preventing that dressing from adhering to the wound.

The good news

On the plus side, contact layer dressings:
- decrease the pain experienced during dressing changes
- can be cut-to-fit or overlap the wound edges.

The not-so-good news

On the minus side, they require a secondary dressing and are contraindicated for use on third-degree burns and infected wounds.

Foam dressings

Foam dressings are spongelike polymer dressings that provide a moist wound environment. These dressings are somewhat absorptive and may include an adhesive border.

Examples of foam dressing include:
- Allevyn Cavity Wound Dressing

- CarraSmart Foam Dressing
- Hydrasorb Foam Wound Dressing
- Mepilex
- PolyTube Tube-Site Dressing
- Tielle Plus Hydropolymer Dressing.

What's the use?

Use a foam dressing as a primary or secondary dressing on wounds with minimal to moderate drainage (including around tubes) when a nonadherent surface is important.

The good news

Here are some advantages of foam dressings:
- Foam dressings with an adhesive border don't require a secondary dressing.
- Foam dressings may be used in combination with other products.
- Hydropolymer foam dressings can manage heavier drainage as they wick moisture from the wound and allow evaporation.

The not-so-good news

Here are some disadvantages:
- Foam dressings may stick to the wound base.
- They can't manage large amounts of drainage.
- They may cause maceration unless they're changed regularly.

Hydrocolloid dressings

Hydrocolloid dressings are adhesive, moldable wafers made of a carbohydrate-based material. Most have a waterproof backing. They're impermeable to oxygen, water, and water vapor, and most hydrocolloid dressings provide some degree of absorption. These dressings turn to gel as they absorb moisture, help maintain a moist wound bed, and promote autolytic debridement.

Examples of hydrocolloid dressings include:
- BandAid Advanced Healing Bandages (available over-the-counter)
- DuoDERM CGF
- Restore Cx Wound Care Dressing
- 3M Tegasorb Hydrocolloid Dressing.

What's the use?

Hydrocolloid dressings should be used for wounds with minimal to moderate drainage, including wounds with necrosis or slough. Hydrocolloid sheet dressings may also be used as secondary dressings.

Hydrocolloid dressings turn to gel as they absorb drainage.

This helps to promote a moist wound bed.

The good news

Hydrocolloid dressings are beneficial because they:
• don't stick to a moist wound base
• maintain moisture by becoming gel as they absorb drainage
• may require changing only two to three times each week
• can be easily removed from the wound base
• are available in contoured forms for use on specific sites
• are available in several varieties (sheets, powder, or gel) in thin and traditional thickness.

The not-so-good news

Some drawbacks of hydrocolloid dressings include that they:
• may have an odor when removed
• can't be used on burns or dry wounds
• can cause skin stripping when removed
• can cause maceration or hypergranulation
• may need to be held in place to maximize adhesion.

Hydrogel dressings

Hydrogel dressings are water- or glycerin-based polymer dressings. They're nonadherent, provide limited absorption (some are 96% water themselves), and come as tubes of gel or in flexible sheets. Hydrogel dressings add moisture and promote autolytic debridement. Examples include:
• Aquasorb Hydrogel Wound Dressing
• Carrasyn Gel Wound Dressing with Acemannan Hydrogel
• CURASOL Gel Wound Dressing
• Hypergel
• Phyto Derma Wound Gel
• SAF-Gel Hydrating Dermal Wound Dressing
• TOE-AID Toe and Nail Dressing.

What's the use?

Hydrogel dressings should be used on dry wounds or wounds with minimal drainage.

The good news

Advantages of hydrogel dressings include that they come in either sheet or amorphous gel form. When applied, they may provide cooling that soothes and eases pain.

The not-so-good news

Disadvantages of hydrogel dressings include that:
• the gel form requires a secondary dressing
• sterile gels are expensive

> Using a hydrogel dressing is like watering a flower bed. The dressing provides moisture to the wound bed.

- viscosity varies among brands and according to the product's base (water or glycerin).

Specialty absorptive dressings

Specialty absorptive dressings have multiple layers of a highly absorbent material, such as cotton or rayon. They may have adhesive borders. Various forms are available, including gels, pads, gauze, or pillows. Examples include:
- AQUACEL
- BreakAway Wound Dressing
- Sofsorb Wound Dressing
- TENDERSORB WET-PRUF Abdominal Pads.

What's the use?

A specialty absorptive dressing should be used on infected or non-infected wounds with heavy drainage.

The good news

The advantages of specialty absorptive dressings are:
- they're highly absorptive
- they require less frequent changes (in most cases)
- they're available in a variety of forms.

The not-so-good news

Specialty absorptive dressings can't be used on burns or on wounds with little or no drainage.

> As their name suggests, specialty absorptive dressings are made for wounds with heavy drainage.

Transparent film dressings

Transparent film dressings are clear, adherent, non-absorptive, polyurethane dressings. They're semipermeable to oxygen and water vapor, but not to water itself. Transparency allows visual inspection of the wound while the dressing is in place. Transparent film dressings maintain a moist wound environment and promote autolysis.

Examples of transparent film dressings include:
- BIOCLUSIVE Transparent Dressing
- BlisterFilm
- ClearSite Transparent Membrane
- OpSite FLEXIGRID
- 3M NexCare Waterproof Bandages (available over-the-counter)
- 3M Tegaderm Transparent Dressing.

What's the use?

Transparent film dressings should be used on partial-thickness wounds with minimal exudate and on wounds with eschar (dry, leathery, black necrotic tissue) to promote autolysis.

The good news

Transparent film dressings:
- may require less frequent changes
- allow you to see the wound without removing the dressing
- are adherent but won't stick to the wound
- aren't bulky.

The not-so-good news

Transparent film dressings don't absorb drainage, so they should be used only on partial-thickness wounds with minimal exudate. In addition, the adhesive border can strip skin when the dressing is removed.

Wound fillers

Wound fillers, as the name suggests, are specialized dressings used to fill deeper wounds. They're made of various materials and come in many forms, such as pastes, granules, powders, beads, and gels. Wound fillers can add moisture to the wound bed or absorb drainage, depending on the product. Examples include:
- AcryDerm STRANDS Absorbent Wound Filler
- Bard Absorption Dressing
- Catrix Wound Dressing
- Multidex Maltodextrin Wound Dressing Gel or Powder.

Wound fillers can go both ways. Some add moisture to the wound bed while others absorb drainage.

What's the use?

Wound filler can be used as a primary dressing on an infected or a noninfected wound with minimal to moderate drainage that requires packing.

The good news

Wound fillers come in various forms and absorptive abilities.

The not-so-good news

Wound fillers can't be used on third-degree burns, on dry wounds, or on wounds with tunnels and sinuses. Also, the wormlike appearance of some wound filler products can alarm a sensitive patient.

Adjunct wound care products

An entire universe of topical skin and wound care aids is available to complement the function of dressings. Because a comprehensive listing would require several companion volumes, we'll limit our discussion to several categories of products and devices that directly impact a wound's ability to heal.

Provant Wound Closure System

The Provant Wound Closure System is a noninvasive treatment that stimulates healing. A treatment signal is directed 2 ¾ to 3 ⅛ (7 to 8 cm) into the tissues around the wound to induce the proliferation of fibroblasts and epithelial cells as well as the secretion of multiple growth factors. The result is faster healing. Treatment doesn't require removal of existing dressings. Clinical studies indicate that the Provant system is effective in promoting healing, even in cases of chronic, severe pressure ulcers.

What's the use?

The Provant system is beneficial to wounds in the inflammatory phase of healing.

The good news

The Provant Wound Closure System:
• requires no special training (patients may be able to perform therapy at home)
• requires only two 30-minute treatments per day (duration is pre-set in the device so it turns off automatically at the end of a session)
• may be used over existing dressings.

The not-so-good news

However, the Provant system:
• can't be used for pregnant patients or those with cardiac pacemakers
• won't help heal bone or deep internal organs.

> The Provant Wound Closure System sends a special signal into the tissues around the wound that keeps me on my toes. The proliferation of fibroblast and epithelial cells means faster healing.

Vacuum-Assisted Closure device

The Vacuum-Assisted Closure (VAC) device uses negative air pressure to promote wound closure. This system consists of a special open-cell polyurethane ether foam dressing cut to the size of the wound, a vacuum tube, and a vacuum pump. One end of the vacuum tube is embedded in the foam dressing and the other connects to the vacuum pump. The dressing is sealed securely in place with adhesive tape that extends 1¼″ to 2″ (3 to 5 cm) over adjacent skin all around the dressing.

When turned on, the pump gently reduces air pressure beneath the dressing, drawing off exudate and reducing edema in surrounding tissues. This process reduces bacterial colonization, promotes granulation tissue development, increases the rate of cell mitosis, and spurs the migration of epithelial cells within the wound. Special training is required to operate this device. (See *Understanding vacuum-assisted closure therapy.*)

The large-capacity VAC device is cumbersome and isn't designed to be moved about. However, a smaller, portable version, called the MiniVAC device, is available. It runs on batteries and has a smaller drainage capacity.

Two new VAC devices have recently been introduced:
• The VAC Freedom device is a portable, lightweight device with a 300-ml drainage capacity.
• The VAC-ATS is ideal for heavily draining wounds for patients in acute care settings. This device has touch-screen operations and a 500-ml drainage capacity.

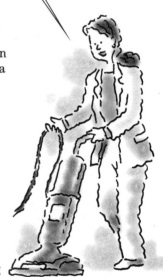

Suck this up! The VAC device aids healing by removing infectious drainage, promoting granulation tissue formation, and drawing wounds closed.

What's the use?

VAC therapy is useful in managing slow-healing acute, subacute, or chronic exudative wounds with cavities. It's ideal for pressure ulcers or surgical wounds with depths greater than 1 cm.

The good news

Here are some advantages of the VAC device:
• It cleans deeply and can manage moderate to large amounts of drainage (VAC drainage capacity is 300 ml; MiniVAC, 50 ml; VAC Freedom, 300 ml; VAC-ATS, 500 ml).
• Dressings can be cut to bridge two or more wounds, permitting one VAC unit to manage multiple wounds.
• The MiniVAC and VAC Freedom have rechargeable batteries and are small enough to fit in pouches that can be worn at the waist or over the shoulder.

The not-so-good news

Here are some disadvantages:
• VAC therapy is contraindicated for use with untreated osteomyelitis, malignancies, or wounds with necrotic tissue or fistulas.
• The VAC vacuum tube is 5′ to 6′ (1.5 to 1.8 m) long, which requires that the patient remain in one place or carry the unit along.
• The VAC and VAC-ATS devices require electricity; the MiniVAC and VAC Freedom batteries must be recharged frequently.

Understanding vacuum-assisted closure therapy

Vacuum-assisted closure (VAC) therapy, also called *negative pressure wound therapy*, is an option to consider when a wound fails to heal in a timely manner. VAC therapy encourages healing by applying localized subatmospheric pressure at the site of the wound. This reduces edema and bacterial colonization and stimulates the formation of granulation tissue.

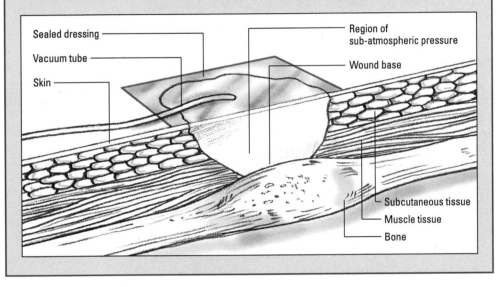

- Sealed dressing
- Vacuum tube
- Skin
- Region of sub-atmospheric pressure
- Wound base
- Subcutaneous tissue
- Muscle tissue
- Bone

- Incorrect use of the VAC device, such as improperly setting the pressure, can result in bruising at the wound base.

Warm-Up Therapy System

The Warm-Up Therapy System for wounds, or noncontact normothermic wound therapy, is a temporary therapy that increases the temperature of the wound bed, thereby promoting increased blood flow in the area of the wound. The dressing in this system contains a special electronic warming card. Once in place, the card heats to 100.4° F (38° C), bathing the wound in radiant heat. The closely sealed wound covering promotes a moist environment in the wound bed. This system is designed to remain in place for 72 hours.

What's the use?

The Warm-Up Therapy System may be used for acute or chronic, full- or partial-thickness wounds, regardless of etiology, that have failed to thrive with traditional therapies, including wounds with compromised blood flow, such as arterial or diabetic foot ulcers.

The good news

The wound covering can absorb a small to moderate amount of drainage.

The not-so-good news

The Warm-Up Therapy System is contraindicated for use on third-degree burns. In addition, it requires specific dressings and thorough patient teaching related to dressing changes and heat management.

Debriding agents

Debriding agents are chemical or enzyme preparations used to debride necrotic or devitalized tissues. These products are applied directly to the offending tissues in the wound. In wounds containing eschar, the eschar is crosshatched so the agent can penetrate the tissue.

Examples of debriding agents include:
- ACCUZYME
- Collagenase Santyl Ointment
- PANAFIL.

What's the use?

These products should be used in debriding wounds with moderate to large amounts of necrotic tissue, especially in cases where surgical debridement isn't an option.

The good news

Some products contain chlorophyll, which helps control odor (drainage may turn green, however, and be wrongly interpreted as infection). Effective debridement requires only a small amount of the agent; more isn't necessarily better.

The not-so-good news

Here are some disadvantages of debriding agents:
- Some ingredients in debriding agents are known allergens.
- Certain debriding agents require secondary dressings.
- Debriding agents can cause irritation if they come in contact with surrounding skin.
- As a debriding agent is applied, it can cause a burning sensation in the wound that can last for several hours.
- Debriding agents are expensive.

> The chlorophyll found in some debriding agents helps to control wound odor.

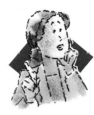

Quick quiz

1. What type of dressing is most appropriate for a patient with a dry wound?

    A.   Specialty absorptive dressing
    B.   Amorphous hydrogel dressing
    C.   Alginate dressing
    D   Foam dressing

Answer: B. A dry wound needs moisture added to promote wound healing, so an amorphous hydrogel dressing should be used.

2. Which dressing type is most absorbent?

    A.   Hydrocolloid
    B.   Foam
    C.   Composite
    D.   Alginate

Answer: D. Although all of these products have some absorptive capacity, alginates are the most absorbent option.

3. What's the advantage of a debriding agent containing chlorophyll?

    A.   It can manage heavy exudate.
    B.   It controls bleeding.
    C.   It controls odor.
    D.   It speeds wound closure.

Answer: C. Chlorophyll helps reduce unpleasant odors.

4. You smell an unpleasant odor as you remove your patient's dressing. Which type of dressing may cause this finding?

    A.   Alginate
    B.   Hydrocolloid
    C.   Composite
    D.   Foam

Answer: B. Hydrocolloid dressings absorb drainage and turn to gel. This gel can have an unpleasant odor when exposed during dressing changes.

5. Which of the following wound care products uses negative air pressure to deep clean a wound?

    A.   VAC device
    B.   Warm-Up Therapy System
    C.   Debriding agent
    D.   Hydrocolloid dressing

Answer: A. The VAC device generates negative pressure that draws off exudate, bacteria, and excessive moisture.

Scoring

☆☆☆ If you answered all five questions correctly, shout it out! Your knowledge of wound care products is second to none.

☆☆ If you answered three or four correctly, we'd like to shake your hand. You've obviously absorbed all the material on wound care products.

☆ If you answered fewer than three questions correctly, that's okay. We'll count this one as warm-up therapy!

Therapeutic modalities

Just the facts

In this chapter, you'll learn:

♦ therapeutic modalities for wound healing

♦ physiologic effects of therapeutic modalities

♦ indications, contraindications, and application methods
  for therapeutic modalities.

A look at therapeutic modalities

Therapeutic modalities have commonly been described as adjunctive modalities—treatments that are used in addition to traditional therapies. Today, this definition is slightly outdated, though, because therapeutic modalities are now part of standard care and are central to the wound healing process. (See *How therapeutic modalities promote healing*, page 196.)

Old meets new

Some therapeutic modalities, such as hydrotherapy and therapeutic light, have been used since the early 1900s. Many traditional modalities are widely used in practice today, and new therapeutic modalities are always in development.

The newest of the new

In many cases, new therapeutic modalities are based on traditional modalities. Some of the newest therapeutic modalities under development involve using near-infrared photo energy, inducing cell proliferation, and delivering ultrasound in a mist.

Selecting a therapeutic modality

To select the best therapeutic modalities for your patient, think about what his wound care needs are.

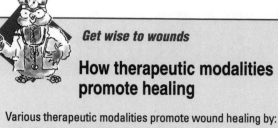

Get wise to wounds

How therapeutic modalities promote healing

Various therapeutic modalities promote wound healing by:
• physically or mechanically debriding particulate and bacterial necrosis
• killing microorganisms or controlling bioburden (microorganism number)
• reducing or controlling edema and wound fluids
• increasing blood flow and tissue oxygenation
• enhancing immune or connective tissue cell function
• providing scaffolding for tissue growth.

Think about your patient's wound care needs. That's the key to selecting the best therapeutic modalities for each patient.

For example...

If the wound needs debridement to remove necrosis and reduce microorganism counts, therapeutic modalities to consider include:
• pulsatile lavage
• whirlpool
• electrical stimulation
• laser therapy
• ultraviolet (UV) treatment (using UVC radiation).

Furthermore...

For edema and lymphedema control and to reduce pathologic intercellular fluid loads, consider:
• electrical stimulation
• compression pumps or stockings.

Finally...

To stimulate tissue formation by increasing blood vessel formation (angiogenesis); enhancing blood flow and the delivery of oxygen, nutrients, and immune cells; facilitating immune cell and wound bed cell function; and stimulating wound matrix formation and collagen fiber alignment, consider:
• growth factors
• living skin equivalents
• pulsatile lavage
• UV treatment (using UVA and UVB radiation)
• ultrasound

- electrical stimulation
- laser therapy
- cell proliferation
- whirlpool.

Common therapeutic modalities

Some of the old and new therapeutic modalities widely embraced by today's wound care practitioners are:
- biotherapy (growth factors, living skin equivalents)
- hydrotherapy (pulsatile lavage, whirlpool)
- therapeutic light (UV treatment, laser therapy)
- ultrasound
- electrical stimulation
- hyperbaric oxygen.

Biotherapy

Two biotherapy methods used in wound treatment include growth factors and living skin equivalents.

Growth factors

Because of the important role that growth factors play in the healing process (stimulating cell proliferation), they're one important form of biotherapy currently used.

A top-notch performance

Wound healing is a complex process that the body undertakes to replace or repair injured tissue. Healing is like a concert performance by an orchestra with many musicians. When everyone knows his part and follows the conductor, the music flows beautifully. However, if one player is out of sync with the rest of the orchestra, the result is a jumbled mixture of noise.

Getting the factors straight

If various growth factors aren't synthesized, secreted, and removed from tissues with correct timing, wound healing becomes jumbled. This leaves the wound bed in a chronic state of confusion, unable to heal.

When wound healing is synchronized, it flows like music from an orchestra...and it has a good beat.

The master factor

In the past decade, growth factors have been studied to determine exactly how they function in healing and how they may be used in the treatment of chronic wounds. Particular focus has been placed on platelet-derived growth factor (PDGF), which some experts call the *master factor*. Although the specific growth factor or other mechanism that initiates wound healing isn't known, PDGF is known to play a central role by attracting fibroblasts and inducing them to divide. This is central to wound healing because fibroblasts are responsible for collagen formation and are one of the components of granulation tissue.

A few more factors

Other key growth factors that play roles in wound healing include:
• transforming growth factor beta (TGF-β) — controls movement of cells to sites of inflammation and stimulates extracellular matrix formation
• basic fibroblast growth factor (bFGF) — stimulates angiogenesis (the development of blood vessels)
• vascular endothelial growth factor (VEGF) — stimulates angiogenesis
• insulin-like growth factor (IGF) — increases collagen synthesis
• epidermal growth factor (EGF) — stimulates epidermal regeneration.

Growth factors on trial

Of these growth factors, PDGF, TGF-β, bFGF, and EGF have been through or are undergoing testing in clinical trials. At this time, the only synthetic growth factor approved for use in wound care is becaplermin (Regranex Gel 0.01%), which has a biological activity similar to that of endogenous PDGF. Regranex increases wound closure by 43%. It's recommended for use on lower-extremity diabetic neuropathic ulcers that have adequate blood flow and involve tissues at and below the subcutaneous level.

A put-on

Regranex can be applied to wounds using a sterile applicator, such as a swab, a tongue blade, or saline-moistened gauze. A dime-size thickness of Regranex is all that's needed. The wound can then be dressed with a saline-moistened gauze.

Living skin equivalents

Another type of biotherapy available for chronic wound management involves the use of living skin equivalents.

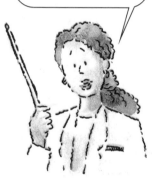

Various growth factors need to be synthesized, secreted, and removed from tissues to optimize wound healing. PDGF is known as the master factor, but it must work with other growth factors for successful wound healing to occur.

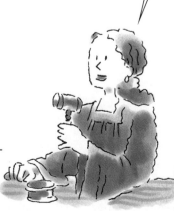

On trial today are the growth factors PDGF, TGF-β, bFGF, and EGF. Only becaplermin — a substance similar to PDGF — has been approved for use in wound care.

Comparing living skin equivalents

Here's how two living skin equivalents measure up to each other.

Product	What it replaces	What it's made from	What it's used for
Dermagraft	Dermis	• Human fibroblasts on a polyglactin mesh	• Burns • Diabetic foot ulcers
Apligraf	Epidermis and dermis	• Type 1 collagen • Human fibroblasts • Human keratinocytes	• Venous ulcers • Diabetic foot ulcers

Living skin equivalents have certain standards of living. The wounds they cover should be free from infection and necrosis and have adequate blood flow.

It's alive!

Living skin equivalents are living constructs derived from biological substances, such as bovine collagen and human neonatal foreskin. Two living skin equivalents approved by the Food and Drug Administration (FDA) in the United States are Dermagraft and graftskin (Apligraf). Dermagraft is used in treating patients with partial-thickness burns and diabetic foot ulcers. Apligraf is approved for use in both venous and diabetic foot ulcers. All living skin equivalents should be used on wounds that are free from infection and necrosis, and have adequate blood flow to support healing. (*Comparing living skin equivalents.*)

One singular solution

Dermagraft is a dermal substitute and, as such, is a single layer composed of human neonatal fibroblasts seeded on a polyglactin mesh (dissolvable suture material). The fibroblasts secrete and fill in this mesh with extracellular matrix.

Dermagraft is contraindicated for use on clinically infected wounds and wounds with sinus tracks and in individuals with known allergies to bovine products.

A two-layered solution

Apligraf is a bilayered skin substitute consisting of an epidermal layer and a dermal layer. The dermal layer is composed of type 1 collagen and human neonatal fibroblasts; the epidermal layer is formed from human keratinocytes (the epidermal cells that synthesize keratin).

When applied to venous ulcers, Apligraf is used along with standard compression therapy. For a patient with diabetic foot ulcers, appropriate off-loading devices are also used.

Contraindications for Apligraf include use on wounds that are infected and use in individuals with known allergies to bovine collagen or other components in the medium in which Apligraf is shipped.

Hydrotherapy

Hydrotherapy, one of the oldest therapeutic modalities, is used in wound care by members of many disciplines.

Getting wet

There are various forms of hydrotherapy, including:
• pulsatile lavage with concurrent suction
• whirlpool therapy
• jet irrigation
• irrigation with a bulb syringe or a syringe with an attached angiocatheter.
As with most treatments, the type of therapy used depends on the patient's wound type.

Pulsatile lavage

Today, most hydrotherapy treatments are delivered by pulsatile lavage. Pulsatile lavage cleans and debrides wounds by combining pulse irrigation with suction.

Advantages of using pulsatile lavage include:
• improved comfort for the patient
• mobility of the apparatus (can be performed in hospital, clinic, or home setting)
• effectiveness in reaching deep, tunneling wounds
• minimized chance of cross-contamination.

Additionally, at least one preliminary study suggests that pulsatile lavage promotes the formation of granulation tissue.

Puttin' on the spritz

Sterile normal saline solution at room temperature is typically used for pulsatile lavage. It's applied by spray gun using a plastic, disposable fan tip. A tunneling tip is used for deep wounds with tunnels or extensive undermining.

The solution is delivered under pressure to the wound bed and concurrently aspirated by negative pressure through a separate plastic tube in the spray gun. The therapist can control both the

> The delivery method of hydrotherapy varies, depending on what type of wound the patient has.

Pressures for pulsatile lavage

The amount of pressure used for pulsatile lavage depends on the patient's wound type:

• High impact and suction pressures are used for dirty, necrotic wounds.

• Intermediate pressures are used for infected wounds.

• Low pressures are used for clean, granulating wounds.

Specific impact, or delivery pressures, and suction pressures are listed below.

Wound type	Impact pressure*	Suction pressure
Clean or granulating	4 to 6 psi	60 to 80 mm Hg
Infected	8 to 10 psi	80 to 100 mm Hg
Necrotic	10 to 12 psi	100 to 120 mm Hg

*Note: Impact pressures less than 15 psi are recommended for wound management. Nonphysician providers shouldn't exceed 15 psi of impact pressure without on-site supervision by a doctor or a specific order for this pressure level.

> Pulsatile lavage is useful in managing many types of wounds, but precautions are prudent to keep the procedure safe.

delivery or impact pressure of the sterile saline and the suction pressure for aspiration of the contaminated fluid. (See *Pressures for pulsatile lavage*.)

Versatility is a virtue

Pulsatile lavage can be used with almost any wound type: acute or chronic, large or small, infected or noninfected, and clean or necrotic.

Indications for pulsatile lavage include:

• clean wounds — to increase granulation tissue formation

• slow-healing wounds — to increase granulation tissue formation

• infected or heavily contaminated wounds — to decrease bioburden levels

• wound bed preparation — for grafting with either skin grafts or living skin equivalents

• removal of necrotic tissue or other particulate.

Pulsatile precautions

Currently, there are no recognized contraindications for pulsatile lavage; however, suggested precautions include:

- using lower impact and suction pressures on fragile tissue
- avoiding direct pressure over exposed nerves and blood vessels
- avoiding high-impact pressure over malignant tissue
- avoiding high-impact and suction pressures and static delivery in areas where excess suction may draw tissue into the tip as well as over grafts and exposed organs and body cavities.

Whirlpool therapy

In whirlpool therapy, part of the body is immersed in a tank of water that has been heated to a prescribed temperature and circulated by an agitator. This therapy softens tissue, removes debris and drainage, and improves blood flow to the area, enhancing the delivery of oxygen and nutrients. Treatment times range from 10 to 20 minutes. A whirlpool tank may also be used for exercise therapy for patients with open wounds or when a therapeutic pool isn't available.

Small, medium, or large

Whirlpool tanks are available in several sizes: small tanks for hands and extremities, medium-sized tanks for lower body treatments, and large tanks for upper and lower body treatments.

Whirlpools are useful for large surface area treatments, especially when these areas are covered with tough necrotic tissue. Whirlpool treatments are useful with painful ulcers when the patient can't tolerate the pressure of a pulsatile lavage head or when allergies to local anesthetics prevent the use of pulsatile lavage.

Tepid, warm, or hot

The temperature ranges used in whirlpool therapy are:
- tepid or nonthermal—80° to 92° F (26.7° to 33.3° C)
- neutral (local skin temperature)—92° to 96° F (35.5° C)
- warm or thermal—96° to 104° F (40° C).

The appropriate water temperature depends on the patient's wound type:
- For *arterial wounds*, a neutral temperature is recommended, along with shorter treatment times (2 to 5 minutes) so as not to increase tissue metabolism in an ischemic limb.
- Tepid whirlpool temperature and short treatment times (2 to 5 minutes) are recommended for venous ulcers because the edema associated with venous ulcers may increase with warm or hot whirlpool for extended treatments due to both heat exposure and the dependent position of the lower extremities.

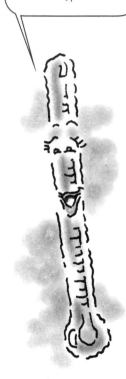

Don't just heat it all the way up! Water temperature in whirlpool therapy varies, depending on the patient's wound type.

Aaah...Now this is what I call hydrotherapy!

• Pressure ulcers and other types of wounds can tolerate neutral to warm temperatures. Warm temperatures may inactivate the harmful enzymes in chronic wound beds.

When to whirl

Indications for whirlpool treatment include:
• large surface area wounds
• wounds with tough, black eschar
• wounds with particulate (such as "road rash")
• painful wounds.

Everybody else, out of the pool!

Contraindications to whirlpool include:
• wound infections
• edema
• deep vein thrombosis or acute phlebitis
• cardiovascular, pulmonary, or renal failure
• unresponsiveness or dementia
• bowel or bladder incontinence
• wounds with dry gangrene.

Therapeutic light

Therapeutic light modalities include UV treatment and laser therapy.

UV treatment

Although not a form of light, UV energy or radiation is commonly categorized as therapeutic light. UV energy lies between X-rays and visible light on the electromagnetic spectrum.

The dawn of light treatment

UV energy has been used for more than 100 years for the treatment of slow healing and infected wounds. Helio-therapy, or sun therapy, has most likely been used since the dawn of humankind for skin problems and other health care needs

3 bands

UV radiation is typically divided into three bands:
- UVA
- UVB
- UVC.

Heliotherapy is as old as the sun.

UVA and UVB benefits

Here are some benefits of treatment with UVA and UVB radiation:
• Chronic pressure ulcers treated with UVA and UVB energy have exhibited increased wound healing in clinical studies.
• UVA and UVB energy enhance white blood cell (WBC) accumulation and lysosomal activity, possibly offering an explanation for UV-mediated debridement.
• UV radiation stimulates the production of interleukin-1 alpha, a cytokine that plays a role in epithelialization.

UVC is a killer

The utility of UVC has been demonstrated in various wound types. It's primarily used for treatment in patients with infected wounds. An added benefit of UVC is that it kills a broad spectrum of microorganisms with low exposure times and isn't likely to generate resistant microorganisms. Recent research has shown that UVC can kill antibiotic-resistant strains of bacteria, such as methicillin-resistant *Staphylococcus aureus*. UVC is easily administered with minimal intervention time and is inexpensive, too. (See *Application of UVC radiation*.)

UV uses

Indications for UV treatment include:
• chronic, slow healing wounds
• infected or heavily contaminated wounds
• necrotic wounds.

Don't use UV

Contraindications for UV treatment include certain chronic disease states, such as:
• diabetes
• pulmonary tuberculosis
• hyperthyroidism
• systemic lupus erythematosus
• cardiac disease
• renal disease
• hepatic disease
• acute eczema
• herpes simplex.

Laser therapy

The word "laser" is actually an acronym for light amplification by stimulated emission of radiation.

Gimme an L! Gimme an A! Gimme an S-E-R! What's that spell? LASER! What's it stand for? Light amplification by stimulated emission of radiation!

Application of UVC radiation

Primarily used to treat patients with infected wounds, ultraviolet C (UVC) radiation kills a broad spectrum of microorganisms with low exposure times. Here's how it's used.

Cover-up

First, the skin around the wound is protected with a thick application of UV-impenetrable ointment, such as zinc oxide or petrolatum. Other skin areas are covered with clean sheets. The eyes of the patient and the person administering the therapy must be covered with UV protective glasses.

Turn-on

The UVC lamp is then placed 1" (2.5 cm) from the surface and then turned on for 30 to 60 seconds. This is done once daily for approximately 1 week or until the infection has cleared. Fungal infections may require a slightly longer treatment time (90 seconds).

Space-out

Tissue spacers, as shown below, may be added to maintain the appropriate distance of the lamp from the wound.

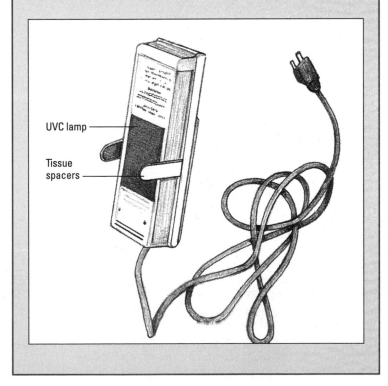

UVC lamp

Tissue spacers

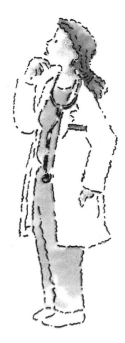

Hot- and cold-running radiation

Lasers can be divided into two groups:
• Cold lasers include the helium neon, or red laser, and the gallium-arsenide laser.
• Hot lasers encompass the carbon dioxide laser and other lasers used for surgical dissection.

In wound healing, cold lasers promote wound closure and nerve regeneration. The treatment consists of either placing the laser probe directly over selected treatment points for a specific time, according to the dose required, or using a gridlike pattern and continuously moving the probe over this grid for a specific treatment time.

Let the laser go

Indications for laser therapy include:
• slow healing wounds
• nerve regeneration
• pain relief.

Lose the laser

Contraindications for laser therapy include treatments over:
• the eye
• a hemorrhage
• a malignancy
• a pregnant woman's uterus
• photosensitive skin.

Ultrasound

Ultrasound (mechanical pressure waves) is used in treatments for patients with both open and closed wounds for its nonthermal and thermal effects.

Nonthermal effects

Nonthermal effects of ultrasound include acoustic cavitation and microstreaming.
• In acoustic cavitation, gaseous bubbles are made to expand and contract rhythmically in the tissues being treated. These bubbles are thought to stimulate biological phenomena, such as the activation of ionic channels in cellular membranes.
• Microstreaming is another nonthermal effect that results from cavitation. Cavitation causes fluids close to the bubbles to stream by, thus stimulating the cells in close proximity. In this

> Ultrasound aids wound healing nonthermally through acoustic cavitation and microstreaming. It's all about bubbles.

way, ultrasound increases calcium conductance in fibroblasts, which is important because collagen secretion is a calcium-dependent process.

Thermal effects

The thermal effects of ultrasound include increasing blood flow, improving migration of WBCs, and promoting an orderly arrangement of collagen.

Ultrasound's thermal effects include increased blood flow to tissue, which results in increased tissue healing. Ultrasound also increases WBC migration and promotes a more orderly arrangement of collagen in both open and closed wounds.

Ultrasound appears to have optimal effects when used early on, during the inflammatory phase of wound healing. It speeds the wound's progress through the healing phases.

Sounds like a job for ultrasound

Ultrasound is indicated to:
- increase wound healing
- enhance blood flow
- decrease pain
- decrease inflammation.

Silence the ultrasound

Contraindications for ultrasound include:
- malignant tissue
- acute infections
- deep vein thrombosis
- ischemic areas
- plastic implants or implanted electronic devices
- irradiated areas
- treatment over the gonads, spinal cord, eyes, or a pregnant woman's uterus.

Electrical stimulation

Electrical stimulation is used to enhance healing of recalcitrant wounds, especially chronic pressure ulcers. The types of electrical stimulation used in wound healing include high-voltage and low-voltage pulsed current. Electrical stimulation is delivered through a device that has conductive electrodes, which are applied to the skin.

Zap it!

Electrical stimulation can be used to:
- orient cells
- promote cellular migration

- enhance blood flow
- increase protein synthesis and wound bed formation
- destroy microorganisms
- provide pain relief.

Electrical stimulation indications

Electrical stimulation is indicated to:
- promote wound healing
- increase blood flow
- increase angiogenesis
- increase tissue oxygenation
- reduce wound bioburden or microbial content
- reduce pain (wound and diabetic neuropathic pain).

Electrical stimulation contraindications

Contraindications for electrical stimulation include:
- malignant tissue
- untreated osteomyelitis
- treatment over pericardial area or areas related to control of cardiac and respiratory function
- treatment over some implanted electronic devices.

Isn't that shocking? High-voltage pulsed current and low-voltage pulsed current are used in wound healing.

Hyperbaric oxygen

Hyperbaric oxygen (HBO) is the delivery of 100% oxygen through a sealed chamber.

In whole or part

Two forms of HBO are used for wound healing. One form involves a total body chamber, such as that used for decompression therapy for divers, and the other involves a smaller chamber used just for the limbs. (The effectiveness of topical HBO through small-limb chambers hasn't yet been proven through research.)

Extra O$_2$

HBO delivered by a whole body chamber increases the amount of dissolved oxygen in the blood that's available for wound healing. This increased availability of readily usable oxygen in the blood provides extra oxygen for use by cells such as neutrophils that employ oxygen-dependent processes. (The processes by which neu-

We have oxygen on our side! Extra oxygen in the blood aids us in battling microorganisms in wounded tissues.

trophils destroy microorganisms are oxygen-based, as is cellular metabolism in general). The increased availability of oxygen for tissues apparently relieves relative hypoxia in wounded tissues.

Evidence supporting systemic or whole body HBO treatment for patients with chronic wounds is evolving. Patients with venous ulcers that don't improve with traditional therapies may benefit when compression therapy is paired with systemic HBO treatment. Another possible use for HBO is in treating patients with diabetic foot ulcers. HBO increases nitric oxide production in the wound. Nitric oxide is a unique free radical that's important in vasodilation and neurotransmission, which play major roles in diabetic wound healing.

When to use HBO

Indications for HBO include:
- diabetic foot ulcers
- venous ulcers.

When to avoid HBO

HBO is contraindicated for:
- patients taking antineoplastic agents
- patients experiencing pneumothorax.

New therapeutic modalities

Several new therapeutic modalities for wound care have evolved in the past decade. Recent developments that are new to the market or haven't yet reached the market are:
- monochromatic near-infrared photo energy (MIRE)
- cell proliferation induction (CPI)
- mist ultrasound transport therapy (MUST).

MIRE without muck

Treatment with MIRE is U.S. FDA-approved for increasing circulation and reducing pain. The nitric oxide that's released into the bloodstream when MIRE is applied to the skin increases blood flow, delivering nutrients to the area and promoting healing. Neural function (sensation) may also improve due to increased blood flow to impaired nerves.

See CPI

CPI technology involves the use of a low-level, confined, radiofrequency signal to stimulate wound healing. The signal is delivered at or near the cycle time for calcium channels, thus inducing the release of growth factors by a calcium-dependent

It's worth repeating: After treatment with MIRE, almost all patients with diabetic neuropathy had improved sensation, possibly due to increased blood flow to impaired nerves.

mechanism. CPI has been shown to increase proliferation of fibroblasts and epithelial cells and has been found to stimulate wound closure in pressure wounds.

MUST is a mist

In MUST, ultrasound energy is transferred directly to the wound through a sterile saline mist. MUST enhances wound healing and decreases bacterial and necrotic debris in tissue by:
- enhancing fibroblast migration rates (shown in the laboratory)
- increasing collagen levels (shown in an animal wound model)
- decreasing bacterial numbers (shown in both the laboratory and a patient case study)
- enhancing blood flow.

The minds, they are a-changin'

These new technologies represent a recent trend in thinking about chronic wound management—that is, that the cells normally involved in wound healing should be stimulated as part of wound care. By doing this, cells are encouraged to do what they do best: orchestrate the complex cascade of events that lead to wound healing.

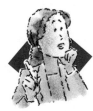

Quick quiz

1. Which of the following growth factors is marketed as Regranex?
    A.   TGF-β
    B.   PDGF
    C.   IGF
    D.   VEGF

Answer: B. Becaplermin (Regranex Gel 0.01%) is the only growth factor substance approved by the FDA for use in wound care. It has a biological activity similar to that of PDGF produced by the body.

2. Which type of hydrotherapy is used most commonly for wound care?
    A.   Pulsatile lavage with concurrent suction
    B.   Whirlpool
    C.   Jet irrigation devices
    D.   Bulb syringe

Answer: A. Today, most hydrotherapy treatments are delivered by pulsatile lavage because of improved comfort for the patient; the mobility of the apparatus; its ability to reach deep, tunneling wounds; the minimal chance for cross-contamination; and the decreased physical and departmental resources required for treatment.

3. What whirlpool temperature should be used for the patient with a venous ulcer?
  A. Cold
  B. Tepid
  C. Warm
  D. Hot

Answer: B. Tepid whirlpool temperature is recommended for venous ulcers because the edema associated with venous ulcers may increase with warm or hot whirlpool temperature. Cold water isn't recommended.

4. What type of UV light is used for infected wounds?
  A. UVA
  B. UVB
  C. UVC
  D. UVD

Answer: C. UVC has been primarily used for the treatment of infected wounds because it kills a broad range of microorganisms with short exposure times. Also, it isn't likely to generate resistant microorganisms.

5. What's the maximum recommended impact pressure for pulsatile lavage?
  A. 5 psi
  B. 10 psi
  C. 15 psi
  D. 20 psi

Answer: C. Unless there's a specific order for a higher impact pressure or a doctor is present to supervise, impact pressure shouldn't exceed 15 psi.

6. Which type of therapy increases the amount of dissolved oxygen in the blood?
  A. Ultrasound
  B. Electrical stimulation
  C. Laser
  D. Hyperbaric oxygen

Answer: D. By increasing the amount of dissolved oxygen in the blood, hyperbaric oxygen therapy increases the availability of oxygen to wounded tissues, which improves healing.

Scoring

☆☆☆   If you answered all six questions correctly, take a bow! You're sizzling hot (like some lasers) when it comes to therapeutic modalities.

☆☆   If you answered four or five questions correctly, don't give up! Time and a quick review will heal your wounded pride.

☆   If you answered fewer than four questions correctly, maybe you whirled through the information too quickly. Review the chapter and try again.

Legal and reimbursement issues

Just the facts

In this chapter, you'll learn:

♦ legal and reimbursement issues related to wound care

♦ established standards for health care practice, including Agency for Healthcare Research and Quality guidelines and state practice acts

♦ documentation strategies that can help you avoid litigation.

A look at legal and reimbursement issues

> Pay close attention to this chapter. The information you find here could keep you out of court.

Wounds affect thousands of people each year. They contribute to morbidity and mortality, increase the cost of care and, sometimes, contribute to liability issues. By learning to properly evaluate wounds, you can dramatically improve your wound care patients' clinical and financial outcomes. At the same time, you'll avoid legal traps and denial of reimbursement.

What's a legal issue?

An *issue* is anything questionable in provided care; it's related to some adverse occurrence or outcome.

The issue is...

Here are some examples of legal issues:
• a possibly negligent action or omission by a health care provider
• deviation from an accepted standard of care
• inconsistencies in documentation.

Question of the day

A common question that comes up in issues of medical malpractice is, "Has the clinician met accepted standards of care?" For example, did a wound care specialist fail to implement preventive measures even though a patient was identified as being at risk for pressure ulcers?

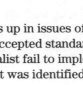

It says here that a standard of care is the level of care, skill, and treatment that's acceptable and appropriate. That seems reasonable.

Standards of care

To safeguard your practice, get to know what standards you're held to in the event of a legal issue.

That's reasonable

Standard of care is a term used to specify what's reasonable under a certain set of circumstances. Standards are used to define certain aspects of a profession, such as the:
- focus of its pursuits
- beneficiaries of service
- responsibilities of its practitioners.
    In health care, the prevailing professional standard of care is defined as the level of care, skill, and treatment deemed acceptable and appropriate by similar health care providers. A standard is a yardstick against which effective care can be measured.

Standard sources

The standards for wound care practice are derived from several sources:
- Agency for Healthcare Research and Quality (AHRQ) guidelines
- Patient's Bill of Rights
- facility- and unit-specific policies and procedures
- job descriptions
- American Nurses Association (ANA) *Standards of Clinical Nursing Practice*
- state nurse practice acts and guidelines.

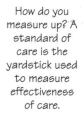

How do you measure up? A standard of care is the yardstick used to measure effectiveness of care.

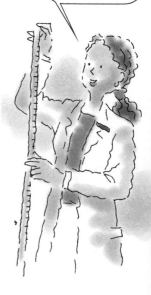

Agency for Healthcare Research and Quality guidelines

Guidelines from the AHRQ—formerly the Agency for Health Care Policy and Research, or AHCPR—are a primary source of wound care standards for all health care practitioners.

What is the AHRQ?

The AHRQ supports research and provides evidence-based information related to health care. (See *Spotlight on the AHRQ.*)

Spotlight on the AHRQ

The Agency for Healthcare Research and Quality (AHRQ) is a federal agency that sponsors and conducts research on major areas of health care, including:

• quality improvement and patient safety
• outcomes and effectiveness of care
• clinical practice and technology assessment
• health care organization and delivery systems
• health care costs and sources of payment.

In the past decade, numerous campaigns have focused on establishing and publishing best-practice guidelines for pressure ulcer prevention and treatment. In the 1990s, the AHCPR sponsored the *Clinical Practice Guidelines* for effective and appropriate care of specific patient populations. Two are specific to wound care:

• *Prevention of Pressure Ulcers* (AHCPR *Clinical Practice Guideline* number 3) deals with tools to identify patients at risk for developing pressure ulcers and guidelines for basic preventive skin care and early treatment.

• *Treatment of Pressure Ulcers* (AHCPR *Clinical Practice Guideline* number 15) provides specific aspects of pressure ulcer care and corresponding evidence to support each recommendation.

Like the *Bill of Rights* that most people are familiar with, the *Patient's Bill of Rights* outlines certain privileges — those related to health care — to which each person is entitled.

Patient's Bill of Rights

The *Patient's Bill of Rights* is another recognized basis for standards of care.

We, the people...

The American Hospital Association first sanctioned a *Patient's Bill of Rights* in 1973 to establish standards of treatment that each patient can expect, including:

• the right to considerate and respectful care
• the right to know, by name, the doctor accountable for his care and to acquire from the doctor thorough information related to his diagnosis, treatment, and prognosis
• the right to receive enough information to give informed consent
• the right to refuse treatment
• the right to privacy relative to his medical care
• the right to confidentiality

- the right to solicit hospital services even if it means evaluation and referral to an accepting hospital
- the right to acquire information such as the names of individuals involved in providing his care
- the right to be informed if the hospital plans to engage in experimental treatment and the right to refuse to partake in such treatment
- the right to expect follow-up care on discharge
- the right to review and receive an explanation of his bill
- the right to understand hospital rules and regulations related to patient conduct.

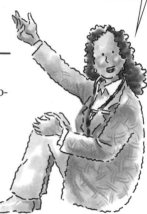

Clinicians are legally obliged to observe and support the *Patient's Bill of Rights* to ensure that patients receive appropriate treatment.

Facility- and unit-specific policies and procedures

The policies and procedures in your facility are also used to establish standards of care.

Mind your Ps and Ps

Policies and procedures are commonly used in litigation claims. Too often, clinicians are informed of policies and procedures but don't take time to examine and understand them. Deviating from facility policies and procedures suggests failure to meet the facility's standards of care.

Job descriptions

Job descriptions are also used to set standards of care.

It *is* your job

How does your employer define the health care team's roles and relationships? Depending on the practice setting—such as hospital, home, or extended care facility—your role may vary.

To protect patients and staff members, firm practice guidelines are needed for all personnel to make sure that job descriptions are accurate. If health care employees practice outside their formal job descriptions, the facility's legal counsel or the insurance company could win a judgment against those employees to recover some of the losses incurred.

Nursing care specialists must live up to high standards established by specialty nursing organizations.

Standards of Clinical Nursing Practice

For professional nursing, the *Standards of Clinical Nursing Practice* outline the expectancy of the comprehensive professional role within which all nurses must practice. Nursing practice standards ensure that the quality of nursing care, documentation, consistency, accountability, and professional credibility are upheld.

Setting the standards

The ANA first published the *Standards of Nursing Practice* in 1973. Since then, specialty nursing organizations have developed their own standards of practice in various areas of nursing, such as in emergency, perioperative, oncologic, and critical care nursing. Some of these standards were developed and published in collaboration with the ANA.

In 1991, the *Standards of Nursing Practice* were revised with participation from state nurses associations and specialty nursing organizations. The revised publication—*Standards of Clinical Nursing Practice*—is a comprehensive outline of expectations for all nurses. *Standards of Clinical Nursing Practice* is composed of authoritative statements describing a level of care or performance common to the nursing profession. It sets a standard by which the quality of nursing practice can be judged.

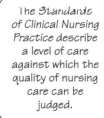

The *Standards of Clinical Nursing Practice* describe a level of care against which the quality of nursing care can be judged.

Setters of wound care standards

The Wound, Ostomy, and Continence Nurses Society (WOCN) is the professional organization for wound, ostomy, and continence (WOC) nurses (formerly known as enterostomal nurses). WOC nurses are experts in skin care and wound management. In 1987, the WOCN standards of care were developed for patients with dermal wounds (pressure sores and leg ulcers). Since then, the standards have been revised to reflect advances in technology and updated research findings.

State nurse practice acts and guidelines

Nurse practice acts and guidelines set by each state are also used to establish standards of care for nurses.

Acts define roles

State nurse practice acts are laws that define which treatments, actions, and functions can be performed or delegated in each state.

For example, conservative sharp debridement is a method of removing loose, nonviable tissue with sterile instruments. According to most state nurse practice acts, it may be performed by "trained healthcare professionals" such as registered nurses. The range of a nurse's legal responsibilities regarding conservative sharp debridement may vary from state to state. It's each nurse's professional responsibility to understand her scope of practice. If a nurse is licensed in more

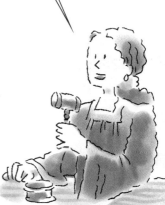

Location is relevant for nurses. A nurse must make sure she's familiar with the guidelines of the state in which she's practicing.

than one state, she needs to make sure that she's familiar with the specific guidelines of the state in which she's practicing.

Litigation

Litigation is a lawsuit that's contested in court to enforce a right or pursue a resolution. Examples of legal liability specifically related to wound care usually involve claims of negligence, such as:
- failure to prevent
- failure to treat
- failure to heal.

Negligence, which is now recognized as a form of malpractice, is defined as failure to meet a standard of care—in other words, failure to do what another reasonably prudent health care provider would do in similar circumstances.

The M word

Clinicians are being sued individually for malpractice with increasing frequency. Malpractice is a health care professional's wrongful conduct, improper discharge of professional duties, or failure to meet standards of care that result in harm to another person. Most malpractice litigation comes as a result of claims that a health care provider failed to:
- provide physical protection
- monitor or assess
- promptly respond
- properly administer a medication.

Practitioners in critical care, emergency, trauma, and obstetrics and those who practice as specialists are most vulnerable.

Merit for medical malpractice

Four criteria must be verified to determine whether a medical malpractice claim is merited:

A *duty* must be established with the patient. What this means is that the clinician accepts accountability for the care and treatment of the patient.

A *breach of duty or standard of care* by the clinician must be determined to evaluate if there has been an act of negligence or breach of duty that resulted in harm to the patient.

Proximate cause or *causal connection* must be established between the breach of duty or standard of care and the damages or injuries to the patient. In other words, the patient must prove that damages were due directly to the clinician's negligence and

> Negligence is considered grounds for a malpractice suit after four criteria are verified.

Memory jogger

To remember the four criteria that merit a medical malpractice claim, think **ABCD**:

Accountability rests with the practitioner.

Breach of duty leads to damages.

Causal connection is established between the breach and the damages.

Damages or injuries are presented as evidence of the breach of duty.

that the damages were foreseeable. In other words, were the damages a direct result of the negligence?

 Damages, or *injuries*, to the patient must be presented as evidence as a result of the alleged negligence. These damages can be physical (disfigurement or pain and suffering), mental (mental anguish), or financial (past, present, or future medical expenses).

If the patient-plaintiff can establish these four components, malpractice litigation is merited.

> Practicing without your own malpractice insurance is risky. The insurance company that covers your employer may be more allegiant to the employer than to you.

Avoiding litigation

The key to reducing your risk of involvement in malpractice litigation is prevention. However, even if you provide optimum care to every patient, there's no guarantee that your actions will never be called into question in a litigation case. If that happens, you must be aware of how you're protected.

A common misconception

Many clinicians practice under the perception that they're protected by their facility's or employer's insurance policy. In most legal claims, your interests and the interests of your employer are comparable. However, the insurance company that provides your employer's coverage may be more allegiant to the employer than to you. In addition, the employer's insurance may not cover you if your performance fell outside your job description or if you didn't follow written policy and procedure.

Practicing without your own malpractice insurance is risky. Malpractice insurance doesn't keep you from getting sued, but it may lift most of the financial burden and fear of a lawsuit off your shoulders. Remember, it's expensive to prove your innocence.

The best defense

Excellent documentation is the key to minimizing your liability. It's direct evidence of your evaluation and care related to wounds. The medical record is your best protection and first line of defense. (See *Documentation do's and don'ts*, page 220.)

At your service

A patient's satisfaction with care also reduces liability. Typically, a malpractice claim represents the connection between patient injury and patient anger. Good communication with the patient and his family is essential to maintaining a good connection.

Documentation do's and don'ts

To protect yourself against liability, document as accurately as possible by following these guidelines.

Do
• Chart factually, specifically, and concisely — Present your observations and interventions clearly and concisely.
• Chart thoroughly — Malpractice claims are commonly filed years later, and the passage of time impairs your ability to remember details. Thorough documentation doesn't lose memories.
• Chart promptly — Making tardy or late entries may lead to inadvertent omissions.

Don't
• Chart personal observations, opinions, feelings, or beliefs — These aspects of care are irrelevant.

Health care is a service industry, so you need to incorporate good customer service into your daily practice, including:
• being respectful and courteous — People become angry when treated rudely.
• being attentive — Give the patients the time that they need.
• being sympathetic and empathetic — Concern pays off in the long run.
• being considerate and honest — Patients recognize honesty, which makes them feel better about the care they receive.
• recognizing your limits — Ask for help or a second opinion if you have doubts.
• staying current — Continuing education is a professional responsibility.

We're here to serve the patients. Make sure you dish up a healthy serving of respectful attention to every customer.

Reimbursement

Understanding finances as they relate to wound care is essential when you're providing care to high-risk patients and those with alterations in skin integrity, such as an ulcer or a wound. Why? Because treating wounds can be costly.

Dollars and sense

With the ever-increasing costs of health care, it's time to recognize your role when it comes to reimbursement. Putting cost-effective wound care into clinical practice requires knowledge of payment systems and documentation strategies.

Payment systems

The language of health insurance is complicated; make sure you can recognize basic terms related to payment systems.

Examples of payment systems include:
- Medicare
- Medicaid
- managed care
- private pay.

Medicare

Medicare is a federal insurance program for people age 65 and older, specific disabled individuals, and people with diagnosed end-stage renal disease. It's administered by the Centers for Medicare and Medicaid Services (CMS).

Medicare A to B

Medicare is split into part A (hospital insurance) and part B (medical insurance):
- Part A coverage encompasses inpatient hospital care, inpatient skilled nursing facility care associated with inpatient hospitalization, home health care after inpatient hospitalization, and hospice care.
- Part B coverage includes services provided by doctors and other health care professionals, ambulance services, and durable medical supplies and equipment (such as wound care dressings and other supplies).

Who pays?

CMS contracts with insurance companies to process and pay claims for health care provided to Medicare beneficiaries. Payment for services and products varies according to practice settings, such as acute care hospitals, skilled nursing facilities, home health care agencies, outpatient facilities, and hospices.

Claims for services and products are submitted using a coding system known as the Healthcare Common Procedure Coding System, or HCPCS. Current Procedural Terminology codes, which are commonly called CPT codes, are used to bill services.

More alphabet soup, please

You may encounter several additional reimbursement terms and acronyms. (See *Recognizing reimbursement terms,* page 222.)

Recognizing reimbursement terms

A veritable alphabet soup of terms is associated with reimbursement for care, services, and products. Being aware of some of these terms can help you keep reimbursement straight.

- Assignment — an agreement in which a provider of services or supplies accepts the approved Medicare amount of payment as payment in full
- BBA — the Balanced Budget Act of 1997, which developed prospective payment systems for Medicare providers
- Capitation — a method of payment whereby an established amount is payable regardless of actual services provided
- CMN — a certificate of medical necessity, which is required by Medicare to document the necessity of medical equipment or supplies
- DRGs — diagnosis related groups, a grouping system used by payment sources for the purpose of classifying inpatient hospital services based on a primary diagnosis, secondary diagnoses, demographics, procedures, and possible complications; the DRG reimbursement compensates services for the entire length of stay
- DME — durable medical equipment, equipment generally used to provide a medical purpose, such as a walker, cane, or vacuum-assisted therapy device
- DMERC — durable medical equipment regional carrier; four regional carriers govern and process Medicare B claims
- OASIS — Outcomes and Assessment Information Set, a required tool for identifying and documenting patient data utilized by Medicare certified home health agencies
- Per Diem Reimbursement — reimbursement that's fixed on a set rate per day
- PPS — prospective payment system, a payment program whereby rates are predetermined and providers are reimbursed regardless of the incurred costs
- RUG — resource utilization groups, a classification system used in nursing facilities to determine a per diem payment rate based on the patient's functional status and acuity
- SNF — skilled nursing facility

Medicaid

Medicaid is a medical assistance program for indigent individuals who are elderly, blind, or disabled and for needy families with dependent children. Although conjointly funded through federal and state regulations, it's administered by state agencies. Reimbursement guidelines vary for each state and in each practice setting.

Managed care

Managed care is a health insurance program that combines benefits presented through Medicare and Medicare Plus Choice. Medicare Plus Choice combines Medicare and private insurance programs—such as health maintenance organizations and preferred provider organizations programs—that may provide benefits not covered by Medicare. Reimbursement is based on fee structures established by each program.

Private pay

Private insurance reimbursement and benefits are also provided in a wide variety of ways. Like the other programs, they have established contracts to pay for services furnished by providers based on reasonable charges. Reasonable charges may include whatever is considered necessary to provide services related to patient care.

Documentation strategies

Health insurance payers are directly involved in treatment decisions because they make decisions regarding payment for medical services and supplies. The fact is, most denials of reimbursement result from insufficient or inconsistent documentation.

Write right

Assessment and documentation are used to determine the patient's care plan and reimbursement decisions. The information used in making care plan and payment decisions comes from the data you provide. Make sure your documentation:
• clearly supports the clinical assessment
• accurately recounts a succession of outcomes related to patient care
• supports payment.

Making progress is imperative

Outcome tracking and reevaluation of the care plan are used to track the healing of a patient's wound. They must be done to avoid reimbursement denial. To maximize reimbursement, the clinician must properly stage and assess wounds and document the patient's progress. Third-party payers no longer pay for continuous wound treatment. They want to see evidence of progress and healing.

> Documentation may seem overwhelming but it's incredibly important. Remember, most reimbursement denials result from insufficient or inconsistent documentation.

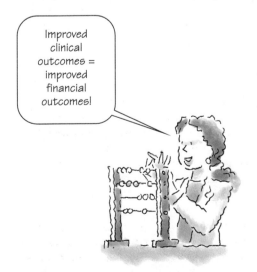

> Improved clinical outcomes = improved financial outcomes!

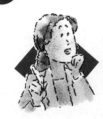

Quick quiz

1. A malpractice suit is brought against a nurse. Her actions will be judged against:
   A.   her state nursing practice act.
   B.   her job description.
   C.   her facility's policies and procedures.
   D.   all of the above.

Answer: D. Standards of care for nurses are established from state nursing practice acts, job descriptions, facility policies and procedures, and other sources. These standards are the measures against which a nurse's actions are judged.

2. Which agency sponsored the development of *Clinical Practice Guidelines* on the prevention and treatment of pressure ulcers?
   A.   CDC
   B.   AHRQ
   C.   NIH
   D.   FDA

Answer: B. The AHRQ, or Agency for Healthcare Research and Quality, is the Federal agency for research on major areas of health care. It sponsored the development of the evidence-based *Clinical Practice Guidelines.*

3. All of the following must be present for a claim of malpractice to be found, except:
   A.   the patient must believe that he has a valid lawsuit.
   B.   a duty must be established.
   C.   a breach of duty or standard must be determined.
   D.   damages or injuries must be presented.

Answer: A. The patient's certainty of having a valid lawsuit isn't enough to merit a malpractice claim. The four components necessary include a duty, breach of that duty, damages or injuries, and causal connection between the breach of duty and the damages.

4. The most effective way you can minimize your liability in a malpractice suit is by:
   A.   charting opinions.
   B.   being disrespectful and discourteous.
   C.   charting accurately, clearly, concisely, promptly, and thoroughly.
   D.   being inattentive.

Answer: C. Accurately charting is your best protection to minimize your liability in a malpractice suit.

5. Implementing cost-effective wound care into clinical practice requires knowledge of:
- A. documentation strategies.
- B. payment systems.
- C. your checkbook balance.
- D. both A and B.

Answer: D. Improved clinical and financial outcomes are directly impacted by the clinician's knowledge of documenting strategies and payment systems.

Scoring

☆☆☆ If you answered all five questions correctly, the ruling is in your favor! You obviously didn't have any issues understanding this chapter.

☆☆ If you answered three or four questions correctly, don't judge yourself too harshly! But do brush up on the information you missed.

☆ If you answered fewer than three questions correctly, just call this a trial run. Prepare to defend yourself next time by reviewing the chapter.

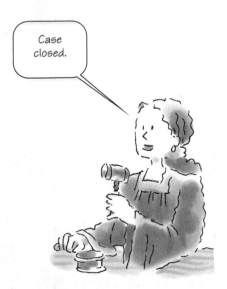

Case closed.

Appendices and index

Pressure ulcer prediction and prevention algorithm

This algorithm, developed by the Agency for Healthcare Policy and Research (now the Agency for Healthcare Research and Quality), can be used to identify patients at risk for pressure ulcers and to prevent pressure ulcer formation. For detailed guidelines, refer to the Clinical Practice Guidelines available online at *www.ahrq.gov/*.

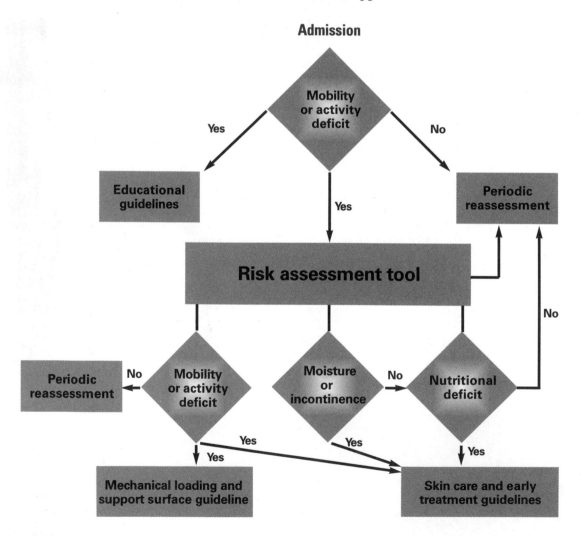

Source: "Pressure Ulcers in Adults: Prediction and Prevention." Clinical Practice Guideline Number 3, AHCPR Publication No. 92-0047: May 1992.

Management of pressure ulcers algorithm

This algorithm, developed by the Agency for Healthcare Policy and Research (now the Agency for Healthcare Research and Quality), can be used to outline the treatment plan for a patient who has a pressure ulcer. For detailed guidelines, refer to the Clinical Practice Guidelines available online at *www.ahrq.gov/*.

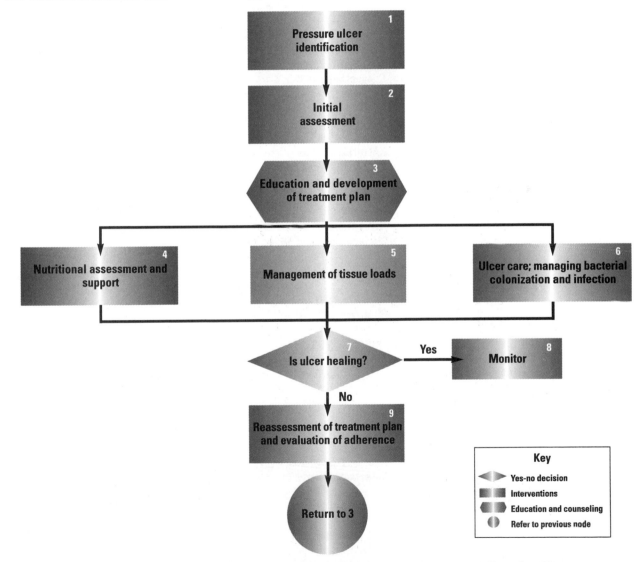

Source: "Pressure Ulcer Treatment." Clinical Practice Guideline Number 15, AHCPR Publication Number 95-0652: December 1994.

Quick guide to wound care dressings

Dressing type	Indications	Products
Alginate	• Wounds with moderate to heavy drainage • Wounds with tunneling	• AlgiCell Calcium Alginate • AlgiDERM Calcium Alginate Dressing or Packing • AlgiSite M • CarboFlex Odor Control Dressing • CarraGinate High G Calcium Alginate Wound Dressing with Acemannan Hydrogel • CarraSorb H Calcium Alginate Wound Dressing • Comfeel Seasorb • Curasorb • Curasorb Zinc • DermaGinate • Hyperion Advanced Alginate Dressing • KALGINATE Calcium Alginate Wound Dressing • KALTOSTAT Wound Dressing • Maxorb CMC/Alginate Dressing • Melgisorb • Restore CalciCare Wound Care Dressing • Sorbsan Topical Wound Dressing • 3M Tegagen HI and HG Alginate Dressings
Biological	• Temporary dressing for skin graft donor sites and burns	• Hyalofill Biopolymeric Wound Dressing • Inerpan Temporary Wound Dressing • Oasis Wound Dressing • Silon Wound Dressing
Collagen	• Chronic, nonhealing, granulated wound beds • Wounds with tunneling	• FIBRACOL PLUS Collagen Wound Dressing with Alginate • Kollagen-Medifil Pads • Kollagen-SkinTemp Sheets
Composite	• Primary or secondary dressing on wounds with light to moderate drainage • Protection for peripheral and central I.V. lines	• Alldress • CompDress Island Dressing • COVADERM PLUS • DuDress Film Top Island Dressing • MPM Multi-Layered Dressing • Repel Wound Dressing • Stratasorb • TELFA Adhesive Dressing • Telfa Island Dressing • TELFA PLUS Island Dressing • 3M Medipore+Pad Soft Cloth Adhesive Wound Dressing

Dressing type	Indications	Products
Composite *(continued)*		• 3M Tegaderm+Pad Transparent Dressing with Absorbent Pad • Viasorb Wound Dressing
Contact layer	• Wounds with minimal, moderate, and heavy drainage; allows for flow of drainage to a secondary dressing while preventing dressing from adhering to the wound	• Conformant 2 Wound Veil • DERMANET Wound Contact Layer • Mepitel • N-TERFACE Interpositional Surfacing Material • Profore Wound Contact Layer • Telfa Clear • 3M Tegapore Wound Contact Material • VersaDress Wound Contact Layer
Foam	• Primary or secondary dressing on wounds with minimal to moderate drainage (including around tubes) when a nonadherent surface is important	• Allevyn and Allevyn Adhesive Hydrophilic Polyurethane Foam Dressing • Allevyn Cavity Wound Dressing • Biatain Adhesive Foam Dressing • Biatain Non-Adhesive Foam Dressing • CarraSmart Foam Dressing • Curafoam Plus Foam Dressing • Curafoam Wound Dressing • EPIGARD • Flexzan Topical Wound Dressing • Hydrasorb Foam Wound Dressing • HydroCell Adhesive Foam Dressing • HydroCell Foam Dressing • HydroCell Thin Adhesive Foam Dressing • LO PROFILE FOAM Wound Dressing • Lyofoam A Polyurethane Foam Dressing • Lyofoam C Polyurethane Foam Dressing with Activated Carbon • Lyofoam Extra Polyurethane Foam Dressing • Lyofoam Polyurethane Foam Dressing • Lyofoam T Polyurethane Foam Dressing • Mepilex • Mepilex Border • Mitraflex • Mitraflex Plus • Odor-Absorbent Dressing • Optifoam Adhesive Foam Island Dressing • Optifoam Non-Adhesive Foam Island Dressing • POLYDERM BORDER Hydrophilic Polyurethane Foam Dressing • Polyderm Hydrophilic Polyurethane Foam Dressing • Polyderm Plus Barrier Foam Dressing • PolyMem Adhesive Cloth Dressings • PolyMem Adhesive Film Dressings • PolyMem Calcium Alginate

Dressing type	Indications	Products
Foam *(continued)*		• PolyMem Non-Adhesive Dressings • PolyTube Tube-Site Dressing • PolyWic Cavity Wound Filler • SOF-FOAM Dressing • SorbaCell Foam Dressing • TIELLE Hydropolymer Adhesive Dressing • TIELLE PLUS Hydropolymer Dressing • VigiFOAM Dressing
Hydrocolloid	• Wounds with minimal to moderate drainage, including wounds with necrosis or slough • Secondary dressings (sheet dressings)	• CarraSmart Hydrocolloid with Acemannan Hydrogel • CombiDERM ACD Absorbent Cover Dressing • CombiDERM Non-Adhesive • Comfeel Paste and Powder • Comfeel Plus Contour Dressing • Comfeel Plus Pressure Relief Dressing • Comfeel Plus Triangle Dressing • Comfeel Plus Ulcer Dressing • Comfeel TRIAD Hydrophilic Wound Dressing • DermaFilm HD • DermaFilm Thin • DERMATELL • DERMATELL SECURE • DuoDERM CGF • DuoDERM CGF Border • DuoDERM Extra Thin • DuoDERM Hydroactive Paste • Exuderm • Exuderm LP • Exuderm RCD • Exuderm Sacrum • Exuderm Ultra • Hydrocol • Hydrocol Sacral • Hydrocol Thin • Hyperion Hydrocolloid Dressing • MPM Excel Hydrocolloid Wound Dressing • PrimaCol Bordered Hydrocolloid Wound Dressing • PrimaCol Hydrocolloid Dressing • PrimaCol Specialty Hydrocolloid Dressing • PrimaCol Thin Hydrocolloid Dressing • Procol Hydrocolloid Dressing • RepliCare • RepliCare Thin • Restore Cx Wound Care Dressing • Restore Extra Thin Dressing

Dressing type	Indications	Products
Hydrocolloid (continued)		• Restore Plus Wound Care Dressing • Restore Wound Care Dressing • SignaDRESS Hydrocolloid Dressing • Sorbex • Sorbexthin • 3M Tegasorb Hydrocolloid Dressings • 3M Tegasorb THIN Hydrocolloid Dressings • Ulcer Care Dressing • Ultec Hydrocolloid Dressing • Ultec Pro Alginate Hydrocolloid Dressing
Hydrogel	• Dry wounds • Wounds with minimal drainage • Wounds with necrosis	• AcryDerm Moist Hydrophilic Wound Dressing • Amerigel Ointment • Aquaflo • AquaGauze Hydrogel Impregnated Gauze Dressing • Aquasite Amorphous Hydrogel • Aquasite Impregnated Gauze Hydrogel • Aquasite Impregnated Non-Woven Hydrogel • Aquasite Sheet Hydrogel • Aquasorb Hydrogel Wound Dressing • Bandage Roll with ClearSite • Biolex Wound Gel • CarraDres Clear Hydrogel Sheet • CarraGauze Pads and Strips with Acemannan Hydrogel • CarraSmart Gel Wound Dressing with Acemannan Hydrogel • Carrasyn Gel Wound Dressing with Acemannan Hydrogel • Carrasyn Spray Gel Wound Dressing with Acemannan Hydrogel • Carrasyn V with Acemannan Hydrogel • Comfort-Aid • Curafil Gel Wound Dressing and Impregnated Strips • Curagel • CURASOL Gel Wound Dressing • DermaGel Hydrogel Sheet • Dermagran Hydrophilic Wound Dressing • Dermagran Zinc-Saline Hydrogel • DermaSyn • DiaB Gel with Acemannan Hydrogel • Elasto-Gel • Elasto-Gel Plus • Elta Hydrogel Impregnated Gauze • Elta Hydrovase Wound Gel • Elta Wound Gel • FlexiGel • Gentell Hydrogel • Hypergel

Dressing type	Indications	Products
Hydrogel *(continued)*		• Hyperion Hydrogel Gauze Dressing • Hyperion Hydrophilic Wound Dressing • Hyperion Hydrophilic Wound Gel • Iamin Hydrating Gel • IntraSite Gel • MPM Excel Gel • MPM GelPad Hydrogel Saturated Dressing • MPM Regenecare • Normlgel • NU-GEL Collagen Wound Gel • PanoGauze Hydrogel Impregnated Gauze Dressing • PanoPlex Hydrogel Wound Dressing • Phyto Derma Wound Gel • Purilon Gel • RadiaGel with Acemannan Hydrogel • RadiaDres Gel Sheet with Acemannan Hydrogel • Restore Hydrogel Dressing • SAF-Gel Hydrating Dermal Wound Dressing • Skintegrity Amorphous Hydrogel • Skintegrity Hydrogel Impregnated Gauze • SoloSite Gel Conformable Wound Dressing • SoloSite Wound Gel • TenderWet Gel Pad • 3M Tegagel Hydrogel Wound Fillers • TOE-AID Toe and Nail Dressing • Ultrex Gel Wound Dressing • Vigilon Primary Wound Dressing • Wound Dressing with ClearSite • WOUN'DRES Collagen Hydrogel
Specialty absorptive	• Infected or noninfected wounds with heavy drainage	• AQUACEL • BAND-AID Brand Island Surgical Dressings • BreakAway Wound Dressing • CombiDERM ACD Absorbent Cover Dressing • CombiDERM Non-Adhesive • Covaderm Adhesive Wound Dressing • CURITY Abdominal Pads • DuPad Abdominal Pads, Open End • DuPad Abdominal Pads, Sealed End • EXU-DRY • Mepore • Multipad Non-Adherent Wound Dressing • Primapore Specialty Absorptive Dressing • Sofsorb Wound Dressing • SURGI-PAD Combine Dressing • TENDERSORB WET-PRUF Abdominal Pads

Dressing type	Indications	Products
Transparent film	• Partial-thickness wounds with minimal exudate • Wounds with eschar	• BIOCLUSIVE Select Transparent Dressing • BIOCLUSIVE Transparent Dressing • Blisterfilm • CarraFilm Transparent Film Dressing • CarraSmart Film Transparent Film Dressing • ClearCell Transparent Film Dressing • ClearSite Transparent Membrane • DERMAVIEW • Mefilm • OpSite • OpSite FLEXIGRID • OpSite PLUS • OpSite Post-Op • Polyskin II Transparent Dressing • Polyskin MR Moisture Responsive Transparent Dressing • ProCyte Transparent Film Dressing • Suresite • 3M Tegaderm HP Transparent Dressing • Transeal Transparent Wound Dressing • UniFlex
Wound filler	• Primary dressing on an infected or a noninfected wound with minimal to moderate drainage that requires packing	• AcryDerm STRANDS Absorbent Wound Filler • Bard Absorption Dressing • CarraSorb M Freeze Dried Gel Wound Dressing with Acemannan Hydrogel • Catrix Wound Dressing • Catrix 5 Rejuvenation Cream • Catrix 10 Ointment • FlexiGel Strands Absorbent Wound Dressing • hyCURE • hyCURE SMART GEL • IODOFLEX PAD • IODOSORB GEL • Kollagen-Medifil II Gel • Kollagen-Medifil II Particles • Multidex Maltodextrin Wound Dressing Gel or Powder

Wound and skin assesment tool

When performing a thorough wound and skin assessment, a pictorial demonstration is often helpful to identify the wound site or sites. Using the wound and skin assessment tool below, the practitioner identified that the left second toe has a partial-thickness vascular ulcer that's red in color.

PATIENT'S NAME (LAST, MIDDLE, FIRST)		ATTENDING PHYSICIAN		ROOM NUMBER	ID NUMBER
Brown, Ann		Dr. A. Dennis		123-2	01726

WOUND ASSESSMENT:

NUMBER	1	2	3	4	5	6
DATE	7/02/03					
TIME	1330					
LOCATION	Ⓛ second toe					
STAGE	II					
APPEARANCE	G					
SIZE-LENGTH	0.5 cm					
SIZE-WIDTH	1 cm					
COLOR/FLR.	R					
DRAINAGE	O					
ODOR	O					
VOLUME	O					
INFLAMMATION	O					
SIZE INFLAM.						

KEY

Stage:
- I. Red or discolored
- II. Skin break/blister
- III. Sub 'Q' tissue
- IV. Muscle and/or bone

Appearance:
- D = Depth
- E = Eschar
- G = Granulation
- IN = Inflammation
- NEC = Necrotic
- PK = Pink
- SL = Slough
- TN = Tunneling
- UND = Undermining
- MX = Mixed (specify)

Color of Wound
Floor:
- RD = Red
- Y = Yellow
- BLK = Black
- MX = Mixed (specify)

Drainage:
- 0 = None
- SR = Serous
- SS = Serosanguinous
- BL = Blood
- PR = Purulent

Odor:
- 0 = None
- MLD = Mild
- FL = Foul

Volume:
- 0 = None
- SC = Scant
- MOD = Moderate
- LG = Large

Inflammation:
- 0 = None
- PK = Pink
- RD = Red

WOUND ANATOMICAL LOCATION:

(cirolc affected area)

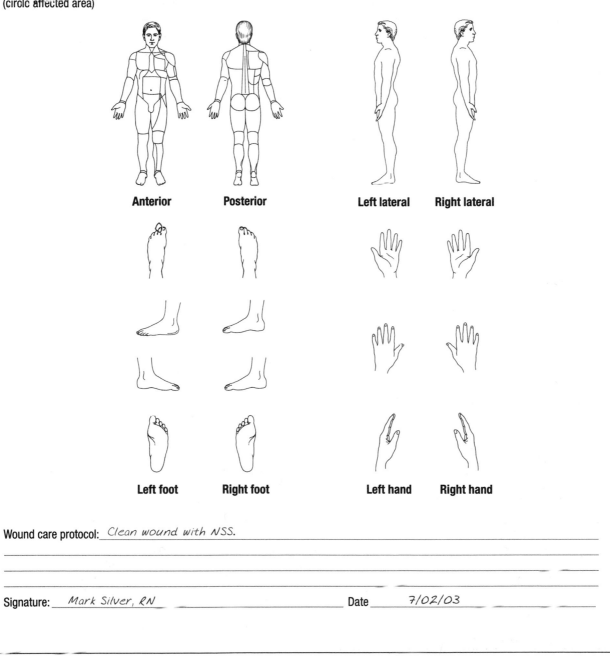

Anterior   **Posterior**   **Left lateral**   **Right lateral**

Left foot   **Right foot**   **Left hand**   **Right hand**

Wound care protocol: _Clean wound with NSS._

Signature: _Mark Silver, RN_   Date _7/02/03_

Using the OASIS B-1 form

If you work in home health care, you may encounter the Outcome and Assessment Information Set (OASIS) form. The latest version, the OASIS-B1, includes more than 80 topics, such as socioeconomic, physiologic, and functional data. The example form here has been filled out with information about a patient with a diabetic foot ulcer.

OUTCOME AND ASSESSMENT INFORMATION SET (OASIS-B1)

START OF CARE Assessment **(also used for Resumption of Care Following Inpatient Stay)**	Client's Name: _____ Client Record No. _____

The Outcome and Assessment Information Set (OASIS) is the intellectual property of The Center for Health Services and Policy Research. Copyright ©2000 Used with Permission.

DEMOGRAPHIC/GENERAL INFORMATION

1. (M0010) Agency Medicare Provider Number:

2. (M0012) Agency Medicaid Provider Number:

5. (M0020) Patient ID Number:
   QCB/811757

6. (M0030) Start of Care Date: 04 / 02 / 2003
   month   day   year

7. (M0032) Resumption of Care Date:
   ___ / ___ / ___   ☒ NA - Not Applicable
   month   day   year

8. (M0040) Patient Name:
   Terry _____ S
   First   MI
   Elliot   Mr.
   Last   Suffix

   Patient Address:
   11 Second Street
   Street, Route, Apt. Number
   Hometown
   City
   (M0050) Patient State of Residence: PA
   (M0060) Patient Zip Code: 10981 - 1234
   Phone: (881) 555 - 2937

9. (M0063) Medicare Number:
   134765482 A
                    including suffix
   ☐ NA - No Medicare

10. (M0064) Social Security Number:
    111 - 22 - 3333
    ☐ UK - Unknown or Not Available

11. (M0065) Medicaid Number:

    ☐ NA - No Medicaid

12. (M0066) Birth Date: 07 / 08 / 1926
    month   day   year

13. (M0069) Gender:
    ☒ 1 - Male   ☐ 2 - Female

14. (M0072) Primary Referring Physician ID:
    222222 _____ (UPIN#)
    ☐ UK - Unknown or Not Available
    Name Dr. Kyle Stevens
    Address 10 State St.
    Hometown, PA 10981
    Phone: (881) 555 - 6900
    FAX: (881) 555 - 6974

15. (M0080) Discipline of Person Completing Assessment:
    ☒ 1-RN   ☐ 2-PT   ☐ 3-SLP/ST   ☐ 4-OT

16. (M0090) Date Assessment Completed:
    04 / 02 / 2003
    month   day   year

17. **(M0100)** This Assessment is Currently Being Completed for the Following Reason:

Start/Resumption of Care

[X] 1 - Start of care — further visits planned

[ ] 2 - Start of care — no further visits planned

[ ] 3 - Resumption of care (after inpatient stay)

Follow-Up

[ ] 4 - Recertification (follow-up) reassessment [Go to *M0150*]

[ ] 5 - Other follow-up [Go to *M0150*]

Transfer to an Inpatient Facility

[ ] 6 - Transferred to an inpatient facility — patient not discharged from agency [Go to *M0150*]

[ ] 7 - Transferred to an inpatient facility — patient discharged from agency [Go to *M0150*]

Discharge from Agency — Not to an Inpatient Facility

[ ] 8 - Death at home [Go to *M0150*]

[ ] 9 - Discharge from agency [Go to *M0150*]

[ ] 10 - Discharge from agency — no visits completed after start/resumption of care assessment [Go to *M0150*]

18. **Marital status:**

[ ] Not Married [X] Married [ ] Widowed
[ ] Divorced [ ] Separated [ ] Unknown

19. **(M0140)** Race/Ethnicity (as identified by patient): (Mark all that apply.)

[ ] 1 - American Indian or Alaska Native

[ ] 2 - Asian

[ ] 3 - Black or African-American

[ ] 4 - Hispanic or Latino

[ ] 5 - Native Hawaiian or Pacific Islander

[X] 6 - White

[ ] UK - Unknown

20. **Emergency contact:**

Name *Susan Elliot*

Address *11 Second St.*

Hometown, PA 10981

Phone: (*881*) *555* - *2937*

21. **(M0150)** Current Payment Sources for Home Care: (Mark all that apply.)

[ ] 0 - None; no charge for current services

[X] 1 - Medicare (traditional fee-for-service)

[ ] 2 - Medicare (HMO/managed care)

[ ] 3 - Medicaid (traditional fee-for-service)

[ ] 4 - Medicaid (HMO/managed care)

[ ] 5 - Workers' compensation

[ ] 6 - Title programs (e.g., Title III, V, or XX)

[ ] 7 - Other government (e.g., CHAMPUS, VA, etc.)

[ ] 8 - Private insurance

[ ] 9 - Private HMO/managed care

[ ] 10 - Self-pay

[ ] 11 - Other (specify) _____

[ ] UK - Unknown

22. **(M0160)** Financial Factors limiting the ability of the patient/family to meet basic health needs: (Mark all that apply.)

[X] 0 - None

[ ] 1 - Unable to afford medicine or medical supplies

[ ] 2 - Unable to afford medical expenses that are not covered by insurance/Medicare (e.g., copayments)

[ ] 3 - Unable to afford rent/utility bills

[ ] 4 - Unable to afford food

[ ] 5 - Other (specify)

PATIENT HISTORY

23. **(M0175)** From which of the following Inpatient Facilities was the patient discharged *during the past 14 days*? (Mark all that apply.)

[ ] 1 - Hospital

[ ] 2 - Rehabilitation facility

[ ] 3 - Skilled nursing facility

[ ] 4 - Other nursing home

[ ] 5 - Other (specify) _____

[X] NA - Patient was not discharged from an inpatient facility [If NA, go to *M0200*]

24. **(M0180)** Inpatient Discharge Date (most recent):

____/____/_____
month day year

[ ] UK - Unknown

(continued)

25. **(M0190)   Inpatient Diagnoses** and ICD code categories (three digits required; five digits optional) *for only those conditions treated during an inpatient facility stay within the last 14 days* (no surgical or V-codes):

Inpatient Facility Diagnosis　　　　　　　　**ICD**

a. _____　　　(_____ . _____)

b. _____　　　(_____ . _____)

26. **(M0200)   Medical or Treatment Regimen Change Within Past 14 Days:** Has this patient experienced a change in medical or treatment regimen (e.g., medication, treatment, or service change due to new or additional diagnosis, etc.) within the last 14 days?

☐ 0 - No   [If No, go to *M0220*]

☒ 1 - Yes

27. **(M0210)** List the patient's **Medical Diagnoses** and ICD code categories (three digits required; five digits optional) or those conditions requiring changed medical or treatment regimen (no surgical or V-codes):

Changed Medical Regimen Diagnosis　　　**ICD**

a. *open wound Ⓛ ankle*　　　　(*891* . *00*)

b. _____　　　(_____ . _____)

c. _____　　　(_____ . _____)

d. _____　　　(_____ . _____)

28. **(M0220)   Conditions Prior to Medical or Treatment Regimen Change or Inpatient Stay Within Past 14 Days:** If this patient experienced an inpatient facility discharge or change in medical or treatment regimen within the past 14 days, indicate any conditions which existed *prior to* the inpatient stay or change in medical or treatment regimen. **(Mark all that apply.)**

☐ 1 - Urinary incontinence

☐ 2 - Indwelling/suprapubic catheter

☐ 3 - Intractable pain

☐ 4 - Impaired decision making

☐ 5 - Disruptive or socially inappropriate behavior

☐ 6 - Memory loss to the extent that supervision required

☒ 7 - None of the above

☐ NA - No inpatient facility discharge *and* no change in medical or treatment regimen in past 14 days

☐ UK - Unknown

29. **(M0230/M0240)   Diagnoses and Severity Index:** List each medical diagnosis or problem for which the patient is receiving home care and ICD code category (three digits required; five digits optional — no surgical or V-codes) and rate them using the following severity index. (Choose one value that represents the most severe rating appropriate for each diagnosis.)

0 - Asymptomatic, no treatment needed at this time

1 - Symptoms well controlled with current therapy

2 - Symptoms controlled with difficulty, affecting daily functioning; patient needs ongoing monitoring

3 - Symptoms poorly controlled, patient needs frequent adjustment in treatment and dose monitoring

4 - Symptoms poorly controlled, history of rehospitalizations

(M0230) Primary Diagnosis　　　　　　　**ICD**

a. _*open wound Ⓛ ankle*_　　　　(*891* . *00*)

Severity Rating ☐ 0   ☐ 1   ☒ 2   ☐ 3   ☐ 4

(M0240) Other Diagnoses　　　　　　　　**ICD**

b. _*Type 2 diabetes*_　　　　　(*250* . *72*)

Severity Rating ☐ 0   ☐ 1   ☒ 2   ☐ 3   ☐ 4

c. _*PVD*_　　　　　　　　　　　(*443* . *89*)

Severity Rating ☐ 0   ☐ 1   ☐ 2   ☒ 3   ☐ 4

d. _____　　(_____ . _____)

Severity Rating ☐ 0   ☐ 1   ☐ 2   ☐ 3   ☐ 4

e. _____　　(_____ . _____)

Severity Rating ☐ 0   ☐ 1   ☐ 2   ☐ 3   ☐ 4

f. _____　　(_____ . _____)

Severity Rating ☐ 0   ☐ 1   ☐ 2   ☐ 3   ☐ 4

30. **Patient/family knowledge and coping level regarding present illness:**

Patient _Knowledgeable about disease process_

Family _Anxious to assist in care_

31. **Significant past health history:** _____

　　　PVD

　　　Type 2 diabetes

　　　Ⓛ BKA

32. **(M0250) Therapies** the patient receives *at home*:
(Mark all that apply.)

- ☐ 1 - Intravenous or infusion therapy (excludes TPN)
- ☐ 2 - Parenteral nutrition (TPN or lipids)
- ☐ 3 - Enteral nutrition (nasogastric, gastrostomy, jejunostomy, or any other artificial entry into the alimentary canal)
- ☒ 4 - None of the above

33. **(M0260) Overall Prognosis:** BEST description of patient's overall prognosis for *recovery from this episode of illness.*

- ☐ 0 - Poor: little or no recovery is expected and/or further decline is imminent
- ☒ 1 - Good/Fair: partial to full recovery is expected
- ☐ UK - Unknown

34. **(M0270) Rehabilitative Prognosis:** BEST description of patient's prognosis for *functional status.*

- ☒ 0 - Guarded: minimal improvement in functional status is expected; decline is possible
- ☐ 1 - Good: marked improvement in functional status is expected
- ☐ UK - Unknown

35. **(M0280) Life Expectancy:** (Physician documentation is not required.)

- ☐ 0 - Life expectancy is greater than 6 months
- ☒ 1 - Life expectancy is 6 months or fewer

36. **Immunization/screening tests:**
Immunizations:

Flu	☒ Yes	☐ No	Date	*10/02*
Tetanus	☒ Yes	☐ No	Date	*3/98*
Pneumonia	☒ Yes	☐ No	Date	*10/02*
Other			Date	

Screening:

Cholesterol level	☒ Yes	☐ No	Date	*11/02*
Mammogram	☐ Yes	☒ No	Date	
Colon cancer screen	☒ Yes	☐ No	Date	*11/02*
Prostate cancer screen	☒ Yes	☐ No	Date	*11/02*

Self-exam frequency:
Breast self-exam frequency
Testicular self-exam frequency

37. **Allergies:** *NKA*

38. **(M0290) High Risk Factors** characterizing this patient: **(Mark all that apply.)**

- ☒ 1 - Heavy smoking
- ☐ 2 - Obesity
- ☐ 3 - Alcohol dependency
- ☐ 4 - Drug dependency
- ☐ 5 - None of the above
- ☐ UK - Unknown

LIVING ARRANGEMENTS

39. **(M0300) Current Residence:**

- ☒ 1 - Patient's owned or rented residence (house, apartment, or mobile home owned or rented by patient/couple/significant other)
- ☐ 2 - Family member's residence
- ☐ 3 - Boarding home or rented room
- ☐ 4 - Board and care or assisted living facility
- ☐ 5 - Other (specify) _____

40. **(M0310) Structural Barriers** in the patient's environment limiting independent mobility: **(Mark all that apply.)**

- ☐ 0 - None
- ☒ 1 - Stairs inside home which *must* be used by the patient (e.g., to get to toileting, sleeping, eating areas)
- ☐ 2 - Stairs inside home which are used optionally (e.g., to get to laundry facilities)
- ☒ 3 - Stairs leading from inside house to outside
- ☐ 4 - Narrow or obstructed doorways

41. **(M0320) Safety Hazards** found in the patient's current place of residence: **(Mark all that apply.)**

- ☒ 0 - None
- ☐ 1 - Inadequate floor, roof, or windows
- ☐ 2 - Inadequate lighting
- ☐ 3 - Unsafe gas/electric appliance
- ☐ 4 - Inadequate heating
- ☐ 5 - Inadequate cooling
- ☐ 6 - Lack of fire safety devices
- ☐ 7 - Unsafe floor coverings
- ☐ 8 - Inadequate stair railings
- ☐ 9 - Improperly stored hazardous materials
- ☐ 10 - Lead-based paint
- ☐ 11 - Other (specify) _____

(continued)

42. **(M0330)** **Sanitation Hazards** found in the patient's current place of residence: (Mark all that apply.)

- [X] 0 - None
- [ ] 1 - No running water
- [ ] 2 - Contaminated water
- [ ] 3 - No toileting facilities
- [ ] 4 - Outdoor toileting facilities only
- [ ] 5 - Inadequate sewage disposal
- [ ] 6 - Inadequate/improper food storage
- [ ] 7 - No food refrigeration
- [ ] 8 - No cooking facilities
- [ ] 9 - Insects/rodents present
- [ ] 10 - No scheduled trash pickup
- [ ] 11 - Cluttered/soiled living area
- [ ] 12 - Other (specify) _____

43. **(M0340)** **Patient Lives With:** (Mark all that apply.)

- [ ] 1 - Lives alone
- [X] 2 - With spouse or significant other
- [ ] 3 - With other family member
- [ ] 4 - With a friend
- [ ] 5 - With paid help (other than home care agency staff)
- [ ] 6 - With other than above

Comments: _____

_____

_____

44. Others living in household: _____

Name _Susan_____ Age _70_ Sex _F_____

Relationship _wife___ Able/willing to assist [X] Yes [ ] No

Name_____ Age_____ Sex_____

Relationship _____ Able/willing to assist [ ] Yes [ ] No

Name_____ Age_____ Sex_____

Relationship _____ Able/willing to assist [ ] Yes [ ] No

Name_____ Age_____ Sex_____

Relationship _____ Able/willing to assist [ ] Yes [ ] No

Name_____ Age_____ Sex_____

Relationship _____ Able/willing to assist [ ] Yes [ ] No

Name_____ Age_____ Sex_____

Relationship _____ Able/willing to assist [ ] Yes [ ] No

SUPPORTIVE ASSISTANCE

45. Persons/Organizations providing assistance:

_____

_____

_____

_____

46. **(M0350)** **Assisting Person(s) Other than Home Care Agency Staff:** (Mark all that apply.)

- [ ] 1 - Relatives, friends, or neighbors living outside the home
- [X] 2 - Person residing in the home (EXCLUDING paid help)
- [ ] 3 - Paid help
- [ ] 4 - None of the above
  [If None of the above, go to *Review of Systems*]
- [ ] UK - Unknown [If Unknown, go to *Review of Systems*]

47. **(M0360)** **Primary Caregiver** taking *lead* responsibility for providing or managing the patient's care, providing the most frequent assistance, etc. (other than home care agency staff):

- [ ] 0 - No one person [If No one person, go to *M0390*]
- [X] 1 - Spouse or significant other
- [ ] 2 - Daughter or son
- [ ] 3 - Other family member
- [ ] 4 - Friend or neighbor or community or church member
- [ ] 5 - Paid help
- [ ] UK - Unknown [If Unknown, go to *M0390*]

48. **(M0370)** **How Often** does the patient receive assistance from the primary caregiver?

- [X] 1 - Several times during day and night
- [ ] 2 - Several times during day
- [ ] 3 - Once daily
- [ ] 4 - Three or more times per week
- [ ] 5 - One to two times per week
- [ ] 6 - Less often than weekly
- [ ] UK - Unknown

49. (M0380) Type of Primary Caregiver Assistance:
(Mark all that apply)

[X] 1 - ADL assistance (e.g., bathing, dressing, toileting, bowel/bladder, eating/feeding)

[X] 2 - IADL assistance (e.g., meds, meals, housekeeping, laundry, telephone, shopping, finances)

☐ 3 - Environmental support (housing, home maintenance)

[X] 4 - Psychosocial support (socialization, companionship, recreation)

[X] 5 - Advocates or facilitates patient's participation in appropriate medical care

☐ 6 - Financial agent, power of attorney, or conservator of finance

☐ 7 - Health care agent, conservator of person, or medical power of attorney

☐ UK - Unknown

Comments: _____

REVIEW OF SYSTEMS

SENSORY STATUS

(Mark S for subjective, O for objectively assessed problem. If no problem present or if not assessed, mark NA.)

Head _N/A_ Dizziness
_N/A_ Headache (describe location, duration) _____

_____

Eyes _O_ Glasses _N/A_ Cataracts _N/A_ Blurred/double vision
_O_ PERRL ____ Other (specify) _____

50. (M0390) Vision with corrective lenses if the patient usually wears them:

[X] 0 - Normal vision: sees adequately in most situations; can see medication labels, newsprint.

☐ 1 - Partially impaired: cannot see medication labels or newsprint, but *can* see obstacles in path, and the surrounding layout; can count fingers at arm's length.

☐ 2 - Severely impaired: cannot locate objects without hearing or touching them *or* patient nonresponsive.

Ears _N/A_ Hearing aid _N/A_ Tinnitus
____ Other (specify) _____

51. (M0400) Hearing and Ability to Understand Spoken Language in patient's own language (with hearing aids if the patient usually uses them):

[X] 0 - No observable impairment. Able to hear and understand complex or detailed instructions and extended or abstract conversation.

☐ 1 - With minimal difficulty, able to hear and understand most multi-step instructions and ordinary conversation. May need occasional repetition, extra time, or louder voice.

☐ 2 - Has moderate difficulty hearing and understanding simple, one-step instructions and brief conversation; needs frequent prompting or assistance.

☐ 3 - Has severe difficulty hearing and understanding simple greetings and short comments. Requires multiple repetitions, restatements, demonstrations, additional time.

☐ 4 - *Unable* to hear and understand familiar words or common expressions consistently, *or* patient nonresponsive.

Oral ____ Gum problems ____ Chewing problems
____ Dentures ____ Other (specify) _____

52. (M0410) Speech and Oral (Verbal) Expression of Language (in patient's own language):

[X] 0 - Expresses complex ideas, feelings, and needs clearly, completely, and easily in all situations with no observable impairment.

☐ 1 - Minimal difficulty in expressing ideas and needs (may take extra time; makes occasional errors in word choice, grammar or speech intelligibility; needs minimal prompting or assistance).

☐ 2 - Expresses simple ideas or needs with moderate difficulty (needs prompting or assistance, errors in word choice, organization, or speech intelligibility). Speaks in phrases or short sentences.

☐ 3 - Has severe difficulty expressing basic ideas or needs and requires maximal assistance or guessing by listener. Speech limited to single words or short phrases.

☐ 4 - *Unable* to express basic needs even with maximal prompting or assistance but is not comatose or unresponsive (e.g., speech is nonsensical or unintelligible).

☐ 5 - Patient nonresponsive or unable to speak.

Nose and sinus
_N/A_ Epistaxis ____ Other (specify) _____

Neck and throat
_N/A_ Hoarseness _N/A_ Difficulty swallowing
____ Other (specify) _____

(continued)

Musculoskeletal, Neurological

N/A Hx arthritis   N/A Joint pain   N/A Syncope

N/A Gout   N/A Weakness   N/A Seizure

N/A Stiffness   S Leg cramps   N/A Tenderness

N/A Swollen joints   S Numbness   N/A Deformities

N/A Unequal grasp   O Temp changes   N/A Comatose

N/A Tremor   N/A Aphasia/inarticulate speech

N/A Paralysis (describe) _____

X Amputation (location) ℝ _below the knee_

___ Other (specify) _____

Coordination, gait, balance (describe) _____

Gait steady

Comments (Prosthesis, appliances) _____

Uses a walker

Patient's perceived pain level: _4_   (Scale 1-10)

53. (M0420) Frequency of Pain interfering with patient's activity or movement:

☐ 0 - Patient has no pain or pain does not interfere with activity or movement

☐ 1 - Less often than daily

☒ 2 - Daily, but not constantly

☐ 3 - All of the time

54. (M0430) Intractable Pain: Is the patient experiencing pain that is *not easily relieved*, occurs at least daily, and affects the patient's sleep, appetite, physical or emotional energy, concentration, personal relationships, emotions, or ability or desire to perform physical activity?

☒ 0 - No

☐ 1 - Yes

Comments (pain management) _____

INTEGUMENTARY STATUS

O Hair changes (where) _Balding_

N/A Puritus   ___ Other (specify) _____

Skin condition (Record type # on body area. Indicate size to right of numbered category.)

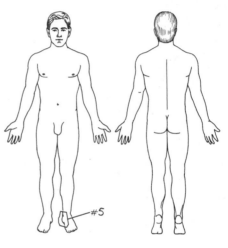

#5

	Type	Size
1.	Lesions	
2.	Bruises	
3.	Masses	
4.	Scars	
5.	Stasis Ulcers	_1/2" round_
6.	Pressure Ulcers	
7.	Incisions	
8.	Other (specify)	

55. (M0440) Does this patient have a Skin Lesion or an Open Wound? This excludes "OSTOMIES."

☐ 0 - No [If No, go to *Cardio/respiratory status*]

☒ 1 - Yes

56. (M0445) Does this patient have a **Pressure Ulcer?**

☒ 0 - No [If No, go to *M0468*]

☐ 1 - Yes

57. (M0450) Current Number of Pressure Ulcers at Each Stage: (Circle one response for each stage.)

Pressure Ulcer Stages	Number of Pressure Ulcers
a) Stage 1: Nonblanchable erythema of intact skin; the heralding of skin ulceration. In darker-pigmented skin, warmth, edema, hardness, or discolored skin may be indicators.	0 1 2 3 4 or more
b) Stage 2: Partial thickness skin loss involving epidermis and/or dermis. The ulcer is superficial and presents clinically as an abrasion, blister, or shallow crater.	0 1 2 3 4 or more
c) Stage 3: Full-thickness skin loss involving damage or necrosis of subcutaneous tissue which may extend down to, but not through, underlying fascia. The ulcer presents clinically as a deep crater with or without undermining of adjacent tissue.	0 1 2 3 4 or more
d) Stage 4: Full-thickness skin loss with extensive destruction, tissue necrosis, or damage to muscle, bone, or supporting structures (e.g., tendon, joint capsule, etc.)	0 1 2 3 4 or more

e) In addition to the above, is there at least one pressure ulcer that cannot be observed due to the presence of eschar or a nonremovable dressing, including casts?

☐ 0 - No
☐ 1 - Yes

58. (M0460) Stage of Most Problematic (Observable) Pressure Ulcer:

☐ 1 - Stage 1
☐ 2 - Stage 2
☐ 3 - Stage 3
☐ 4 - Stage 4
☐ NA - No observable pressure ulcer

59. (M0464) Status of Most Problematic (Observable) Pressure Ulcer:

☐ 1 - Fully granulating
☐ 2 - Early/partial granulation
☐ 3 - Not healing
☐ NA - No observable pressure ulcer

60. (M0468) Does this patient have a Stasis Ulcer?

☐ 0 - No [If No, go to M0482]
☒ 1 - Yes

61. (M0470) Current Number of Observable Stasis Ulcer(s):

☐ 0 - Zero
☒ 1 - One
☐ 2 - Two
☐ 3 - Three
☐ 4 - Four or more

62. (M0474) Does this patient have at least one Stasis Ulcer that Cannot be Observed due to the presence of a nonremovable dressing?

☒ 0 - No
☐ 1 - Yes

63. (M0476) Status of Most Problematic (Observable) Stasis Ulcer:

☐ 1 - Fully granulating
☒ 2 - Early/partial granulation
☐ 3 - Not healing
☐ NA - No observable stasis ulcer

64. (M0482) Does this patient have a Surgical Wound?

☒ 0 - No [If No, go to Cardio/Respiratory Status]
☐ 1 - Yes

65. (M0484) Current Number of (Observable) Surgical Wounds: (If a wound is partially closed but has more than one opening, consider each opening as a separate wound.)

☐ 0 - Zero
☐ 1 - One
☐ 2 - Two
☐ 3 - Three
☐ 4 - Four or more

66. (M0486) Does this patient have at least one Surgical Wound that Cannot be Observed due to the presence of a nonremovable dressing?

☐ 0 - No
☐ 1 - Yes

67. (M0488) Status of Most Problematic (Observable) Surgical Wound:

☐ 1 - Fully granulating
☐ 2 - Early/partial granulation
☐ 3 - Not healing
☐ NA - No observable surgical wound

(continued)

CARDIO/RESPIRATORY STATUS

Temperature _99_   Respirations _18_

Blood pressure
  Lying _132/80_   Sitting _130/78_   Standing _130/76_

Pulse
  Apical rate _72_   Radial rate _72_
  Rhythm _Regular_   Quality _____

Cardiovascular
  _N/A_ Palpitations   _N/A_ Chest pains
  _S_ Claudication   _N/A_ Murmurs
  _S_ Fatigues easily   _O_ Edema
  _N/A_ BP problems   _N/A_ Cyanosis
  _N/A_ Dyspnea on exertion   _N/A_ Varicosities
  _N/A_ Paroxysmal nocturnal dyspnea
  _N/A_ Orthopnea (# of pillows)
  _N/A_ Cardiac problems (specify) _____
  _N/A_ Pacemaker _____
                (Date of last battery change)
  Other (specify) _____
  Comments _____
  _____
  _____

Respiratory
  History of
  _N/A_ Asthma   _N/A_ Pleurisy
  _N/A_ TB   _N/A_ Pneumonia
  _S_ Bronchitis   _N/A_ Emphysema
  Other (specify) _____
  Present condition
  _S_ Cough (describe) _Dry_
  _O_ Breath sounds (describe) _Clear_
  _N/A_ Sputum (character and amount) _____
  Other (specify) _____

68. **(M0490)** When is the patient dyspneic or noticeably **Short of Breath**?

  ☒ 0 - Never, patient is not short of breath

  ☐ 1 - When walking more than 20 feet, climbing stairs

  ☐ 2 - With moderate exertion (e.g., while dressing, using commode or bed-pan, walking distances less than 20 feet)

  ☐ 3 - With minimal exertion (e.g., while eating, talking, or performing other ADLs) or with agitation

  ☐ 4 - At rest (during day or night)

69. **(M0500)** Respiratory Treatments utilized at home:
    (Mark all that apply.)

  ☐ 1 - Oxygen (intermittent or continuous)

  ☐ 2 - Ventilator (continually or at night)

  ☐ 3 - Continuous positive airway pressure

  ☒ 4 - None of the above

  Comments _____
  _____
  _____
  _____

ELIMINATION STATUS

Genitourinary Tract
  _N/A_ Frequency   _N/A_ Prostate disorder
  _N/A_ Pain   _N/A_ Dysmenorrhea
  _N/A_ Hematuria   _N/A_ Lesions
  _N/A_ Vaginal discharge/bleeding _N/A_ Hx hysterectomy
  _S_ Nocturia   _N/A_ Gravida/Para
  _N/A_ Urgency   _N/A_ Contraception
  _N/A_ Date last PAP _____
  Other (specify) _____

70. **(M0510)** Has this patient been treated for a **Urinary Tract Infection** in the past 14 days?

  ☒ 0 - No

  ☐ 1 - Yes

  ☐ NA - Patient on prophylactic treatment

  ☐ UK - Unknown

71. **(M0520)** Urinary Incontinence or Urinary Catheter Presence:

  ☒ 0 - No incontinence or catheter (includes anuria or ostomy for urinary drainage) [If No, go to _M0540_]

  ☐ 1 - Patient is incontinent

  ☐ 2 - Patient requires a urinary catheter (i.e., external, indwelling, intermittent, suprapubic) [Go to _M0540_]

72. **(M0530) When** does **Urinary Incontinence** occur?

☐ 0 - Timed-voiding defers incontinence

☐ 1 - During the night only

☐ 2 - During the day and night

Comments (e.g., appliances and care, bladder programs, catheter type, frequency of irrigation and change) _____

_____

_____

_____

_____

Gastrointestinal Tract

N/A Indigestion   *N/A* Rectal bleeding

N/A Nausea/vomiting   *N/A* Hemorrhoids

N/A Ulcers   *N/A* Gallbladder problems

N/A Pain   *N/A* Jaundice

N/A Diarrhea/constipation *N/A* Tenderness

N/A Hernias (where) _____ _____

Other (specify) _____

73. **(M0540) Bowel Incontinence Frequency:**

☒ 0 - Very rarely or never has bowel incontinence

☐ 1 - Less than once weekly

☐ 2 - One to three times weekly

☐ 3 - Four to six times weekly

☐ 4 - On a daily basis

☐ 5 - More often than once daily

☐ NA - Patient has ostomy for bowel elimination

☐ UK - Unknown

74. **(M0550) Ostomy for Bowel Elimination:** Does this patient have an ostomy for bowel elimination that (within the last 14 days):

a) was related to an inpatient facility stay, *or*

b) necessitated a change in medical or treatment regimen?

☒ 0 - Patient does *not* have an ostomy for bowel elimination.

☐ 1 - Patient's ostomy was *not* related to an inpatient stay and did *not* necessitate change in medical or treatment regimen.

☐ 2 - The ostomy *was* related to an inpatient stay or *did* necessitate change in medical or treatment regimen.

Comments (bowel function, stool color, bowel program, GI series, abd. girth) _____

_____

_____

Nutritional status

N/A Weight lose/gain last 3 mos. (Give amount _____)

N/A Over/under weight   *N/A* Change in appetite

Diet *20% protein 30% fat* _____

Other (specify) _____

Meals prepared by *Wife* _____

Comments _____

_____

_____

_____

_____

Breasts (For both male and female)

N/A Lumps   *N/A* Tenderness

N/A Discharge   *N/A* Pain

Other (specify) _____

Comments _____

_____

_____

NEURO/EMOTIONAL/BEHAVIORAL STATUS

N/A Hx of previous psych. illness

Other (specify) _____

75. **(M0560) Cognitive Functioning:** (Patient's current level of alertness, orientation, comprehension, concentration, and immediate memory for simple commands.)

☐ 0 - Alert/oriented, able to focus and shift attention, comprehends and recalls task directions independently.

☒ 1 - Requires prompting (cueing, repetition, reminders) only under stressful or unfamiliar conditions.

☐ 2 - Requires assistance and some direction in specific situations (e.g., on all tasks involving shifting of attention), or consistently requires low stimulus environment due to distractibility.

☐ 3 - Requires considerable assistance in routine situations. Is not alert and oriented or is unable to shift attention and recall directions more than half the time.

☐ 4 - Totally dependent due to disturbances such as constant disorientation, coma, persistent vegetative state, or delirium.

(continued)

76. (M0570) When Confused (Reported or Observed):

☒ 0 - Never

☐ 1 - In new or complex situations only

☐ 2 - On awakening or at night only

☐ 3 - During the day and evening, but not constantly

☐ 4 - Constantly

☐ NA - Patient nonresponsive

77. (M0580) When Anxious (Reported or Observed):

☐ 0 - None of the time

☐ 1 - Less often than daily

☒ 2 - Daily, but not constantly

☐ 3 - All of the time

☐ NA - Patient nonresponsive

78. (M0590) Depressive Feelings Reported or Observed in Patient: (Mark all that apply.)

☐ 1 - Depressed mood (e.g., feeling sad, tearful)

☐ 2 - Sense of failure or self-reproach

☒ 3 - Hopelessness

☐ 4 - Recurrent thoughts of death

☐ 5 - Thoughts of suicide

☐ 6 - None of the above feelings observed or reported

79. (M0600) Patient Behaviors (Reported or Observed): (Mark all that apply.)

☐ 1 - Indecisiveness, lack of concentration

☐ 2 - Diminished interest in most activities

☐ 3 - Sleep disturbances

☐ 4 - Recent change in appetite or weight

☐ 5 - Agitation

☐ 6 - A suicide attempt

☒ 7 - None of the above behaviors observed or reported

80. (M0610) Behaviors Demonstrated *at Least Once a Week* (Reported or Observed): (Mark all that apply.)

☐ 1 - Memory deficit: failure to recognize familiar persons/places, inability to recall events of past 24 hours, significant memory loss so that supervision is required

☐ 2 - Impaired decision making: failure to perform usual ADLs or IADLs, inability to appropriately stop activities, jeopardizes safety through actions

☐ 3 - Verbal disruption: yelling, threatening, excessive profanity, sexual references, etc.

☐ 4 - Physical aggression: aggressive or combative to self and others (e.g., hits self, throws objects, punches, dangerous maneuvers with wheelchair or other objects)

☐ 5 - Disruptive, infantile, or socially inappropriate behavior (**excludes** verbal actions)

☐ 6 - Delusional, hallucinatory, or paranoid behavior

☒ 7 - None of the above behaviors demonstrated

81. (M0620) Frequency of Behavior Problems (Reported or Observed) (e.g., wandering episodes, self-abuse, verbal disruption, physical aggression, etc.):

☒ 0 - Never

☐ 1 - Less than once a month

☐ 2 - Once a month

☐ 3 - Several times each month

☐ 4 - Several times a week

☐ 5 - At least daily

82. (M0630) Is this patient receiving **Psychiatric Nursing Services** at home provided by a qualified psychiatric nurse?

☒ 0 - No

☐ 1 - Yes

Comments _____

_____

_____

Endocrine and hematopoietic

S   Diabetes   NA Polydipsia

NA Polyuria   NA Thyroid problem

NA Excessive bleeding or bruising

S   Intolerance to heat and cold

Fractionals

Usual results_____

Frequency checked _____

Other (specify) _____

Comments _____

ADL/IADLs

For M0640-M0800, complete the "Current" column for all patients. For these same items, complete the "Prior" column only at start of care and at resumption of care; mark the level that corresponds to the patient's condition 14 days prior to start of care date (M0030) or resumption of care date (M0032). In all cases, record what the patient is *able to do.*

83. (M0640) Grooming: Ability to tend to personal hygiene needs (i.e., washing face and hands, hair care, shaving or makeup, teeth or denture care, fingernail care).

Prior   Current

[X]   ☐   0 - Able to groom self unaided, with or without the use of assistive devices or adapted methods.

☐   [X]   1 - Grooming utensils must be placed within reach before able to complete grooming activities.

☐   ☐   2 - Someone must assist the patient to groom self.

☐   ☐   3 - Patient depends entirely upon someone else for grooming needs.

☐   UK - Unknown

84. (M0650) Ability to Dress *Upper* Body (with or without dressing aids) including undergarments, pullovers, front-opening shirts and blouses, managing zippers, buttons, and snaps:

Prior   Current

[X]   ☐   0 - Able to get clothes out of closets and drawers, put them on and remove them from the upper body without assistance.

☐   [X]   1 - Able to dress upper body without assistance if clothing is laid out or handed to the patient.

☐   ☐   2 - Someone must help the patient put on upper body clothing.

☐   ☐   3 - Patient depends entirely upon another person to dress the upper body.

☐   UK - Unknown

85. (M0660) Ability to Dress *Lower* Body (with or without dressing aids) including undergarments, slacks, socks or nylons, shoes:

Prior   Current

[X]   ☐   0 - Able to obtain, put on, and remove clothing and shoes without assistance.

☐   ☐   1 - Able to dress lower body without assistance if clothing and shoes are laid out or handed to the patient.

☐   [X]   2 - Someone must help the patient put on undergarments, slacks, socks or nylons, and shoes.

☐   ☐   3 - Patient depends entirely upon another person to dress lower body.

☐   UK - Unknown

86. (M0670) Bathing: Ability to wash entire body. *Excludes* grooming (washing face and hands only).

Prior   Current

☐   ☐   0 - Able to bathe self in s*hower or tub* independently.

[X]   ☐   1 - With the use of devices, is able to bathe self in shower or tub independently.

☐   ☐   2 - Able to bathe in shower or tub with the assistance of another person:
(a) for intermittent supervision or encouragement or reminders, *OR*
(b) to get in and out of the shower or tub, *OR*
(c) for washing difficult-to-reach areas.

☐   [X]   3 - Participates in bathing self in shower or tub, *but* requires presence of another person throughout the bath for assistance or supervision.

☐   ☐   4 - *Unable* to use the shower or tub and is bathed in *bed or bedside chair.*

☐   ☐   5 - Unable to effectively participate in bathing and is totally bathed by another person.

☐   UK - Unknown

87. (M0680) Toileting: Ability to get to and from the toilet or bedside commode.

Prior   Current

[X]   [X]   0 - Able to get to and from the toilet independently with or without a device.

☐   ☐   1 - When reminded, assisted, or supervised by another person, able to get to and from the toilet.

☐   ☐   2 - *Unable* to get to and from the toilet but is able to use a bedside commode (with or without assistance).

☐   ☐   3 - *Unable* to get to and from the toilet or bedside commode but is able to use a bedpan/urinal independently.

☐   ☐   4 - Is totally dependent in toileting.

☐   UK - Unknown

(continued)

88. (M0690)　Transferring: Ability to move from bed to chair, on and off toilet or commode, into and out of tub or shower, and ability to turn and position self in bed if patient is bedfast.

Prior　Current

☐　☐　0 - Able to independently transfer.

☒　☒　1 - Transfers with minimal human assistance or with use of an assistive device.

☐　☐　2 - *Unable* to transfer self but is able to bear weight and pivot during the transfer process.

☐　☐　3 - Unable to transfer self and is *unable* to bear weight or pivot when transferred by another person.

☐　☐　4 - Bedfast, unable to transfer but is able to turn and position self in bed.

☐　☐　5 - Bedfast, unable to transfer and is *unable* to turn and position self.

☐　　　UK - Unknown

89. (M0700)　Ambulation/Locomotion: Ability to *SAFELY* walk, once in a standing position, or use a wheelchair, once in a seated position, on a variety of surfaces.

Prior　Current

☒　☐　0 - Able to independently walk on even and uneven surfaces and climb stairs with or without railings (i.e., needs no human assistance or assistive device).

☐　☒　1 - Requires use of a device (e.g., cane, walker) to walk alone or requires human supervision or assistance to negotiate stairs or steps or uneven surfaces.

☐　☐　2 - Able to walk only with the supervision or assistance of another person at all times.

☐　☐　3 - Chairfast, *unable* to ambulate but is able to wheel self independently.

☐　☐　4 - Chairfast, unable to ambulate and is *unable* to wheel self.

☐　☐　5 - Bedfast, unable to ambulate or be up in a chair.

☐　　　UK - Unknown

90. (M0710)　Feeding or Eating: Ability to feed self meals and snacks. **Note: This refers only to the process of** *eating, chewing,* **and** *swallowing, not preparing* **the food to be eaten.**

Prior　Current

☒　☒　0 - Able to independently feed self.

☐　☐　1 - Able to feed self independently but requires:
　　　　(a) meal set-up; *OR*
　　　　(b) intermittent assistance or supervision from another person; *OR*
　　　　(c) a liquid, pureed or ground meat diet.

☐　☐　2 - *Unable* to feed self and must be assisted or supervised throughout the meal/snack.

☐　☐　3 - Able to take in nutrients orally *and* receives supplemental nutrients through a nasogastric tube or gastrostomy.

☐　☐　4 - *Unable* to take in nutrients orally and is fed nutrients through a nasogastric tube or gastrostomy.

☐　☐　5 - Unable to take in nutrients orally or by tube feeding.

☐　　　UK - Unknown

91. (M0720)　Planning and Preparing Light Meals (e.g., cereal, sandwich) or reheat delivered meals:

Prior　Current

☒　☐　0 - (a) Able to independently plan and prepare all light meals for self or reheat delivered meals; OR
　　　　(b) Is physically, cognitively, and mentally able to prepare light meals on a regular basis but has not routinely performed light meal preparation in the past (i.e., prior to this home care admission).

☐　☒　1 - *Unable* to prepare light meals on a regular basis due to physical, cognitive, or mental limitations.

☐　☐　2 - Unable to prepare any light meals or reheat any delivered meals.

☐　　　UK - Unknown

92. (M0730)　Transportation: Physical and mental ability to *safely* use a car, taxi, or public transportation (bus, train, subway).

Prior　Current

☐　☐　0 - Able to independently drive a regular or adapted car; OR uses a regular or handicap-accessible public bus.

☒　☒　1 - Able to ride in a car only when driven by another person; OR able to use a bus or handicap van only when assisted or accompanied by another person.

☐　☐　2 - Unable to ride in a car, taxi, bus, or van, and requires transportation by ambulance.

☐　　　UK - Unknown

93. (M0740) Laundry: Ability to do own laundry—to carry laundry to and from washing machine, to use washer and dryer, to wash small items by hand.

Prior   Current

☐   ☐   0 - (a) Able to independently take care of all laundry tasks; *OR*

          (b) Physically, cognitively, and mentally able to do laundry and access facilities, but has not routinely performed laundry tasks in the past (i.e., prior to this home care admission).

☒   ☐   1 - Able to do only light laundry, such as minor hand wash or light washer loads. Due to physical, cognitive, or mental limitations, needs assistance with heavy laundry such as carrying large loads of laundry.

☐   ☒   2 - *Unable* to do any laundry due to physical limitation or needs continual supervision and assistance due to cognitive or mental limitation.

☐   UK - Unknown

94. (M0750) Housekeeping: Ability to safely and effectively perform light house-keeping and heavier cleaning tasks.

Prior   Current

☐   ☐   0 - (a) Able to independently perform all housekeeping tasks; *OR*

          (b) Physically, cognitively, and mentally able to perform *all* housekeeping tasks but has not routinely participated in housekeeping tasks in the past (i.e., prior to this home care admission).

☐   ☐   1 - Able to perform only *light* housekeeping (e.g., dusting, wiping kitchen counters) tasks independently.

☐   ☐   2 - Able to perform housekeeping tasks with intermittent assistance or supervision from another person.

☐   ☐   3 - *Unable* to consistently perform any housekeeping tasks unless assisted by another person throughout the process.

☒   ☒   4 - Unable to effectively participate in any housekeeping tasks.

☐   UK - Unknown

95. (M0760) Shopping: Ability to plan for, select, and purchase items in a store and to carry them home or arrange delivery.

Prior   Current

☐   ☐   0 - (a) Able to plan for shopping needs and independently perform shopping tasks, including carrying packages; *OR*

          (b) Physically, cognitively, and mentally able to take care of shopping, but has not done shopping in the past (i.e., prior to this home care admission).

☐   ☐   1 - Able to go shopping, but needs some assistance:

          (a) By self is able to do only light shopping and carry small packages, but needs someone to do occasional major shopping; *OR*

          (b) *Unable* to go shopping alone, but can go with someone to assist.

☒   ☒   2 - *Unable* to go shopping, but is able to identify items needed, place orders, and arrange home delivery.

☐   ☐   3 - Needs someone to do all shopping and errands.

☐   UK - Unknown

96. (M0770) Ability to Use Telephone: Ability to answer the phone, dial numbers, and *effectively* use the telephone to communicate.

Prior   Current

☒   ☒   0 - Able to dial numbers and answer calls appropriately and as desired.

☐   ☐   1 - Able to use a specially adapted telephone (i.e., large numbers on the dial, teletype phone for the deaf) and call essential numbers.

☐   ☐   2 - Able to answer the telephone and carry on a normal conversation but has difficulty with placing calls.

☐   ☐   3 - Able to answer the telephone only some of the time or is able to carry on only a limited conversation.

☐   ☐   4 - *Unable* to answer the telephone at all but can listen if assisted with equipment.

☐   ☐   5 - Totally unable to use the telephone.

☐   ☐   NA - Patient does not have a telephone.

☐   UK - Unknown

MEDICATIONS

97. (M0780) Management of Oral Medications: *Patient's ability* to prepare and take all prescribed oral medications reliably and safely, including administration of the correct dosage at the appropriate times/intervals. *Excludes injectable and I.V. medications.* (NOTE: This refers to ability, not compliance or willingness.)

Prior   Current

☒   ☒   0 - Able to independently take the correct oral medication(s) and proper dosage(s) at the correct times.

☐   ☐   1 - Able to take medication(s) at the correct times if:

          (a) individual dosages are prepared in advance by another person; *OR*

          (b) given daily reminders; *OR*

          (c) someone develops a drug diary or chart.

☐   ☐   2 - *Unable* to take medication unless administered by someone else.

☐   ☐   NA - No oral medications prescribed.

☐   UK - Unknown

(continued)

98. (M0790) Management of Inhalant/Mist Medications:
Patient's ability to prepare and take all prescribed inhalant/mist medications (nebulizers, metered dose devices) reliably and safely, including administration of the correct dosage at the appropriate times/intervals. *Excludes* all other forms of medication (oral tablets, injectable and I.V. medications).

Prior Current

☐ ☐ 0 - Able to independently take the correct medication and proper dosage at the correct times.

☐ ☐ 1 - Able to take medication at the correct times if:
    (a) individual dosages are prepared in advance by another person, *OR*
    (b) given daily reminders.

☐ ☐ 2 - *Unable* to take medication unless administered by someone else.

☒ ☒ NA - No inhalant/mist medications prescribed.

☐ UK - Unknown

99. (M0800) Management of Injectable Medications: *Patient's ability* to prepare and take all prescribed injectable medications reliably and safely, including administration of correct dosage at the appropriate times/intervals. *Excludes* I.V. medications.

Prior Current

☒ ☒ 0 - Able to independently take the correct medication and proper dosage at the correct times.

☐ ☐ 1 - Able to take injectable medication at correct times if:
    (a) individual syringes are prepared in advance by another person, OR
    (b) given daily reminders.

☐ ☐ 2 - Unable to take injectable medications unless administered by someone else.

☐ ☐ NA - No injectable medications prescribed.

☐ UK - Unknown

EQUIPMENT MANAGEMENT

100. (M0810) Patient Management of Equipment (includes *ONLY* oxygen, I.V./infusion therapy, enteral/parenteral nutrition equipment or supplies): *Patient's ability* to set up, monitor and change equipment reliably, and safely add appropriate fluids or medication, clean/store/dispose of equipment or supplies using proper technique. (NOTE: This refers to ability, not compliance or willingness.)

☐ 0 - Patient manages all tasks related to equipment completely independently.

☐ 1 - If someone else sets up equipment (i.e., fills portable oxygen tank, provides patient with prepared solutions), patient is able to manage all other aspects of equipment.

☐ 2 - Patient requires considerable assistance from another person to manage equipment, but independently completes portions of the task.

☐ 3 - Patient is only able to monitor equipment (e.g., liter flow, fluid in bag) and must call someone else to manage the equipment.

☐ 4 - Patient is completely dependent on someone else to manage all equipment.

☒ NA - No equipment of this type used in care [If NA, go to *M0825*]

101. (M0820) Caregiver Management of Equipment (includes *ONLY* oxygen, I.V./infusion equipment, enteral/parenteral nutrition, ventilator therapy equipment or supplies): *Caregiver's ability* to set up, monitor, and change equipment reliably and safely, add appropriate fluids or medication, clean/store/dispose of equipment or supplies using proper technique. (NOTE: This refers to ability, not compliance or willingness.)

☐ 0 - Caregiver manages all tasks related to equipment completely independently.

☐ 1 - If someone else sets up equipment, caregiver is able to manage all other aspects.

☐ 2 - Caregiver requires considerable assistance from another person to manage equipment, but independently completes significant portions of task.

☐ 3 - Caregiver is only able to complete small portions of task (e.g., administer nebulizer treatment, clean/store/dispose of equipment or supplies).

☐ 4 - Caregiver is completely dependent on someone else to manage all equipment.

☐ NA - No caregiver

☐ UK - Unknown

THERAPY NEED

102. (M0825) Therapy Need: Does the care plan of the Medicare payment period for which this assessment will define a case mix group indicate a need for therapy (physical, occupational, or speech therapy) that meets the threshold for a Medicare high-therapy case mix group?

☐ 0 - No

☐ 1 - Yes

☐ NA - Not applicable

EQUIPMENT AND SUPPLIES

Equipment needs (check appropriate box)

Has	Needs	
☐	☐	Oxygen/Respiratory Equip.
☐	☐	Wheelchair
☐	☐	Hospital Bed
☒	☐	Other (specify) _Walker_

Supplies needed and comments regarding equipment needs

Financial problems/needs

SAFETY

Safety measures recommended to protect patient from injury

NA

Emergency plans

Wife will call 911 for emergency care if needed.

CONCLUSIONS

Conclusions/impressions and skilled interventions performed this visit

Wound care performed per plan of care. Initiated teaching regarding wound care signs & symptoms of wound infection and emergency measures.

Date of assessment *4/2/03*

Signature of Assessor *Holly Dougherty, RN, BSN*

Glossary

abrasion
a wearing away of the skin through some mechanical process, such as friction or trauma

abscess
a circumscribed collection of pus that forms in tissue as a result of acute or chronic localized infection and is associated with tissue destruction and, in many cases, swelling

acute wound
any wound that's new or progressing as expected

albumin
a large protein molecule that's water-soluble and provides colloid osmotic pressure

alginate
a nonwoven, highly absorptive dressing that's manufactured from seaweed (kelp)

angiogenesis
the formation and regeneration of blood vessels

antimicrobial
an agent that kills microbes or inhibits their growth

autolysis
the breakdown of tissues or cells by the body's own mechanisms, such as enzymes or white blood cells

bacteria
one-celled microorganisms that break down dead tissue, have no true nucleus, and reproduce by cell division

blanchable erythema
a reddened area of the skin that temporarily turns white or pale when pressure is applied with a fingertip; also known as reactive hyperemia

bottoming out
flattening of the support surface of the body, determined by the caregiver placing an outstretched hand (palm up) under the mattress overlay, below the part of the body at risk for ulcer formation (if the caregiver feels that the support material is less than 1-inch thick at this site, the patient has "bottomed out")

burn
an acute wound that's caused by exposure to thermal extremes, caustic chemicals, electricity, or radiation

cellulitis
cellular or connective tissue inflammation that's characterized by redness, swelling, and tenderness

chemical debridement
the topical application of biologic enzymes to breakdown devitalized tissue

chronic wound
any wound that isn't healing in a timely fashion (healing has slowed or stopped)

collagen
the main supportive protein of skin, tendon, bone, cartilage, and connective tissue

colloid osmotic pressure
the force that prevents fluid from leaking out of blood vessels into nearby tissues

colonized
contaminated with bacteria

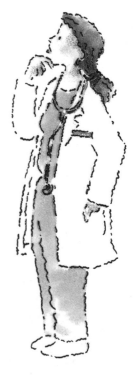

contamination
the presence of bacteria, microorganisms, or other foreign material in or on tissues (wounds with bacterial counts of 10 or fewer organisms per gram of tissue are usually considered contaminated; those with higher counts are generally considered infected)

cytotoxic agents
compounds that destroy both diseased and healthy cells that may be used to clean wounds; examples include povidone-iodine, Dakin's solution, and hydrogen peroxide

dead space
an area of tissue destruction or loss that extends out from main body of wound, leaving a cavity or tract (this area is lightly packed to avoid superficial closure that can lead to abscess formation)

debridement
the removal of necrotic (dead) tissue to allow underlying healthy tissue to regenerate

debris
the remains of broken down or damaged cells or tissue

dehiscence
a partial or total separation of skin and tissue layers

demyelination
the destruction of a nerve's myelin sheath, which interferes with normal nerve conduction

dermis
the thick, inner layer of skin

diabetes mellitus
a metabolic disorder characterized by hyperglycemia resulting from lack of insulin, lack of insulin effect, or both

differentiation
the remodeling of collagen from a gel-like consistency to a mature scar (this maturation imparts mechanical strength to the tissue)

drainage
the fluid produced by a wound, which may contain serum, cellular debris, bacteria, leukocytes, pus, or blood

enzyme
a protein that acts as a catalyst to induce chemical changes in other substances.

epidermis
the outermost layer of skin

epithelialization
the regeneration of epidermis across the wound surface

erythema
an inflammatory redness of the skin caused by engorged capillaries

eschar
nonviable (dead) wound tissue that's characterized by a dry, leathery, black crust

evisceration
the abrupt protrusion of underlying visceral organs from a wound

excoriation
abrasions or scratches on the skin

exudate
any fluid that has been extruded from tissue or capillaries, usually due to injury or inflammation; it's characteristically high in protein and white blood cells

fascia
a band of white fibrous tissue that lies deep in relation to the skin and forms a supportive sheath for muscles and various body organs

fibrin
an insoluble protein that's formed from fibrinogen by the proteolytic action of thrombin and is essential in blood clotting

fibroblasts
the most common cells in connective tissue; responsible for making fibers and extracellular matrix, which provides support to cells

fistula
an abnormal passage between two organs or between an organ and the skin

foam
a spongelike polymer dressing that may or may not be adherent, may be impregnated or coated with other materials, and has some absorptive properties

friction
the act of rubbing one surface against another; may lead to the physiologic wearing away of tissue

full-thickness wound
any wound that penetrates completely through the skin into underlying tissues; adipose tissue, muscle, tendon, or bone may be exposed

gauze
a woven cotton or synthetic fabric dressing that's absorptive and permeable to water, water vapor, and oxygen and may be impregnated with petrolatum, antiseptics, or other agents

granulation
the formation of soft, pink, fleshy projections during the healing process in a wound not healing by primary intention, consisting of new capillaries surrounded by fibrous collagen; tissue appears reddened from the rich blood supply

healing ridge
a buildup of collagen fibers that begins to form during the inflammatory phase of wound healing and peaks during the proliferation phase

hemorrhage
bleeding (may be internal or external)

hydrocolloid
an adhesive, moldable wafer dressing that's made of carbohydrates, has a nonpermeable waterproof backing, and may have some absorptive properties

hydrogel
a water-based nonadherent dressing that has some absorptive qualities

hydrophilic
the ability to readily absorb moisture

hypoxia
the reduction of oxygen in body tissues to below normal levels

induration
tissue firmness that may occur around a wound margin following blanchable erythema or chronic venous congestion

infection
a pathogenic contamination that's reacted against but can't be controlled by the body's immune system

inflammation
a localized protective response elicited by injury or destruction of tissue that's characterized by heat, redness, swelling, pain, and loss of function.

insulin
a hormone secreted into the blood by the islets of Langerhans of the pancreas that promotes the storage of glucose, among other functions

irrigation
cleaning tissue and removing cell debris and drainage from an open wound by flushing it with a stream of liquid

ischemia
deficient blood supply to a body organ or tissue

lymphedema
the chronic swelling of a body part from accumulation of interstitial fluid secondary to obstruction of lymphatic vessels or lymph nodes

maceration
the softening of a solid as it's soaked in fluid (in wounds, maceration is indicated by whitened tissue)

macrophage
a highly phagocytic cell that's stimulated by inflammation

mechanical debridement
the removal of foreign material and devitalized or contaminated tissue from a wound by physical force rather than by chemical (enzymatic) or natural (autolytic) forces; examples include wet-to-dry dressings, wound irrigation, and whirlpool therapy

melanin
a dark skin pigment that filters ultraviolet radiation and is produced and dispersed by specialized cells called *melanocytes*

myelin
a lipidlike substance that surrounds the axon of myelinated nerve fibers and permits normal neurologic conduction

necrosis
cell or tissue death

neuron
a highly specialized conductor cell that receives and transmits electrochemical nerve impulses

neutrophil
a type of white blood cell that's responsible for phagocytosis

nonblanching erythema
a redness of the skin that persists when gentle pressure is applied to it and released

nutritional assessment
an assessment of the relationship between nutrients consumed and energy expended, especially when illness or surgery compromises a patient's intake or alters his metabolic requirements (includes a dietary history, physical assessment, anthropometric measurements, and diagnostic tests)

partial-thickness wound
any wound that involves only the epidermal layer of the skin, or extends through the epidermis and into—but not through—the dermis

pathogen
any microorganism capable of producing disease

peripheral vascular disease
a group of disorders that affect the blood vessels outside the heart or the lymphatic vessels

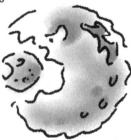

phagocyte
a cell that ingests microorganisms, other cells, and foreign particles

phagocytosis
the engulfment of microorganisms, other cells, and foreign particles by a phagocyte

polyneuropathy
damage to multiple types of nerves

pressure
a force that's applied vertically or perpendicular to a surface

pressure gradient
the difference in pressure between two points (the transmission of pressure from one tissue to another causes an increase in pressure to those tissues that are deepest)

pressure ulcers
wounds that are the clinical manifestation of localized tissue death due to lack of blood flow in areas under pressure

primary dressing
a dressing that's placed directly on the wound bed

protein
a large, complex molecule composed of amino acids, which are essential for tissue growth and repair

pus
a thick, yellowish fluid that's composed of albuminous substances, thin fluid, and leukocytes

reactive hyperemia
an increased amount of blood in a body part following stoppage and subsequent restoration of the blood supply

sebaceous gland
a saclike structure that produces sebum

sebum
a fatty substance that lubricates and softens the skin

sharp debridement
the removal of foreign material or devitalized (dead) tissue using a sharp instrument such as a scalpel

shearing force
a mechanical force that runs parallel, rather than perpendicular, to an area of skin (deep tissues feel the brunt of this force)

sinus tract
a cavity or channel that permits the drainage of wound contents

skin sealant
a clear liquid that creates a film barrier to seal and protect the skin from trauma

slough
nonviable tissue that's loosely attached; characterized by stringlike, moist, necrotic debris; and yellow, green, or gray in color

subcutaneous tissue
a layer of loose connective tissue below the epidermis and dermis that contains major blood vessels, lymph vessels, and nerves; also known as the *hypodermis*

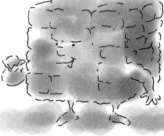

surgical wound
a healthy and uncomplicated break in the skin's continuity resulting from surgery

tendon
a fibrous cord of connective tissue that attaches the muscle to bone or cartilage and enables bones to move when skeletal muscles contract

tensile strength
the maximum force or pressure that can be applied to a wound without causing it to break apart

tissue
a large group of individual cells that perform a certain function

tissue biopsy
the use of a sharp instrument to obtain a sample of skin, muscle, or bone for diagnostic purposes

transparent film
a clear, adherent, nonabsorptive dressing that's permeable to oxygen and water vapor

traumatic wound
a sudden, unplanned injury to the skin that can range from minor to severe

tunnel
an extension of the wound bed into adjacent tissue; also known as *sinus tract*

undermining
a tunneling effect or pocket under the edges of a wound that's caused by the pressure gradient transmitted from the body surface to the bone

vascular wound
any chronic wound that stems from peripheral vascular disease in the venous, arterial, or lymphatic system

wet-to-dry dressing
a dressing that's used in debridement; gauze moistened with normal saline solution is applied to the wound and then removed once the gauze becomes dry and adheres to the wound bed

wound
any break in the skin

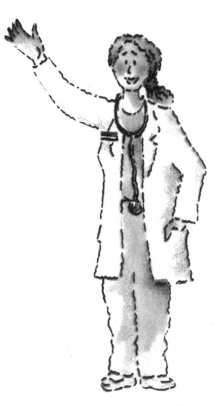

Selected references

Baranoski, S., and Salcido, R. "Seizing the Opportunities for Wound Healing," *Advances in Skin and Wound Care* 15(2):93, March-April 2002.

Baxter, H. "How a Discipline Came of Age: A History of Wound Care," *Journal of Wound Care* 11(10):383-86, 388, 390, November 2002.

Bowker, J.H., and Pfiefer, M.A, eds. *Levin and O'Neal's The Diabetic Foot*, 6th ed. St. Louis: Mosby–Year Book, Inc., 2001.

Bryant, R.A., ed. *Acute and Chronic Wounds: Nursing Management*, 2nd ed. St. Louis: Mosby–Year Book, Inc., 2000.

Corral, O.L., et al. "Wound-Care Resources on the Internet: An Update," *Journal of the American Podiatric Medical Association* 92(9):524-27, October 2002.

Cullen, B., and Parry, G. "Merging Roles: A Successful Approach to Wound Care in the Home," *Caring* 21(6): 14-16, June 2002.

Fishman, T.D. "Wound Assessment and Evaluation," *Dermatology Nursing* 13(1):59-60, February 2001.

Glover, D. "Making Progress on Our Pledge to 'Inform the World About Wound Care,'" *Journal of Wound Care* 11(7): 242-43, July 2002.

Hall, P. and Schumann, L. "Wound Care: Meeting the Challenge," *Journal of the American Academy of Nurse Practitioners* 13(6):258-66, June 2001.

Hess, C.T. "Assessing a Fistula, Part 1," *Nursing2002* 32(8):22, August 2002.

Hess, C.T. *Clinical Guide to Wound Care*, 4th ed. Springhouse, Pa.: Springhouse Corp., 2002.

Hess, C.T. "Management of a Diabetic Foot Ulcer," *Advances in Skin and Wound Care* 14(1):18, January-February 2001.

Hess, C.T. "Management of a Venous Ulcer: A Case Study Approach," *Advances in Skin and Wound Care* 14(3):148-49, May-June 2001.

Kinsella, A. "Advanced Telecare for Wound Care Delivery," *Home Healthcare Nurse* 20(7):457-61, July 2002.

Krasner, D.L. "How to Prepare the Wound Bed," *Ostomy/Wound Management* 47(4):59-61, April 2001.

Macdonald, J.M. "Wound Healing and Lymphedema: A New Look at an Old Problem," *Ostomy/Wound Management* 47(4):52-57, April 2001.

Maklebust, J., and Sieggreen, M. *Pressure Ulcers: Guidelines for Prevention and Management*, 3rd ed. Springhouse, Pa.: Springhouse Corp., 2000.

Margolis, D.J., et al. "Diabetic Neuropathic Foot Ulcers: The Association of Wound Size, Wound Duration, and Wound Grade on Healing," *Diabetes Care* 25(10):1835-39, October 2002.

Orsted, H.L., et al. "Chronic Wound Caring...A Long Journey Toward Healing," *Ostomy/Wound Management* 47(10):26-36, October 2001.

Ovington, L.G. "Battling Bacteria in Wound Care," *Home Healthcare Nurse* 19(10):622-30, October 2001.

Ovington, L.G. "Hanging Wet-to-Dry Dressings Out to Dry," *Home Healthcare Nurse* 19(8):477-83, August 2001.

Ovington, L.G. "Wound Care Products: How to Choose," *Advances in Skin and Wound Care* 14(5):259-64, September-October 2001.

Pattison, P.S. "The Importance of Reassessment to Chronic Wound Care," *Ostomy/Wound Management* 47(8):24-25, August 2001.

Pompeo, M.Q. "The Role of 'Wound Burden' in Determining the Costs Associated with Wound Care," *Ostomy/Wound Management* 47(3):65-71, March 2001.

Salcido, R. "The Point of Education in Wound Care," *Advances in Skin and Wound Care* 14(1):6, January-February 2001.

Salcido, R.S. "It Takes a Village: The Caregiver's Role in Wound Care," *Advances in Skin and Wound Care* 14(5):220, 222, September-October 2001.

Schaum, K.D. "Documentation of Wound Exudate Amount Leads to Dressing Reimbursement after Discharge," *Home Healthcare Nurse* 20(6):399, June 2002.

Schaum, K.D. "Medicare Documentation Guidelines for Wound Care Nurses," *Advances in Skin and Wound Care* 15(3):142-43, May-June 2002.

Schaum, K.D. "Unscramble the Alphabet Soup of Medicare Payment Systems," *Advances in Skin and Wound Care* 14(4):176-78, July-August 2001.

Sussman, C., and Bates-Jensen, B., eds. *Wound Care: A Collaborative Practice Manual for Physical Therapists and Nurses*, 2nd ed. Gaithersburg, Md.: Aspen Pubs., Inc., 2001.

Watts, S.A. "Platelet-Derived Growth Factor for Foot Ulcerations: An Effective Adjunct to Good Wound Care," *Advance for Nurse Practitioners* 9(9):60-63, September 2001.

Wientjes, K.A. "Mind-Body Techniques in Wound Healing," *Ostomy/Wound Management* 48(11):62-67, November 2002.

Wysocki, A.B. "Evaluating and Managing Open Skin Wounds: Colonization Versus Infection," *AACN Clinical Issues* 13(3):382-97, August 2002.

Index

i refers to an illustration; t refers to a table; bold numbers refer to color pages.

i refers to an illustration; t refers to a table; bold numbers refer to color pages.

i refers to an illustration; t refers to a table; bold numbers refer to color pages.

i refers to an illustration; t refers to a table; bold numbers refer to color pages.

i refers to an illustration; t refers to a table; bold numbers refer to color pages.

i refers to an illustration; t refers to a table; bold numbers refer to color pages.

i refers to an illustration; t refers to a table; bold numbers refer to color pages.

i refers to an illustration; t refers to a table; bold numbers refer to color pages.

i refers to an illustration; t refers to a table; bold numbers refer to color pages.

i refers to an illustration; t refers to a table; bold numbers refer to color pages.

i refers to an illustration; t refers to a table; bold numbers refer to color pages.

XY

Z

i refers to an illustration; t refers to a table; bold numbers refer to color pages.

Notes

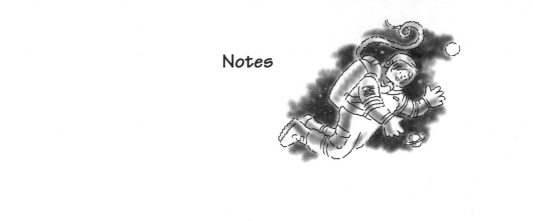

Notes

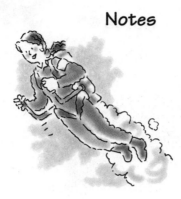

Notes

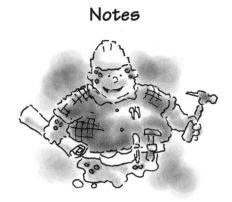

Notes

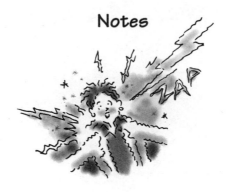